DO NOT REMOVE
CARDS FROM POCKET

ALLEN COUNTY PUBLIC LIBRARY

FORT WAYNE, INDIANA 46802

You may return this book to any agency, branch,
or bookmobile of the Allen County Public Library.

STDs: Sexually Transmitted Diseases

What You Should Know and How to Protect Yourself

by
STEPHEN H. ZINNER, M.D.

Professor of Medicine and Chief, Division of
Infectious Diseases, Department of Medicine,
Brown University and Roger Williams
General Hospital

SUMMIT BOOKS   NEW YORK

Copyright © 1985 by Stephen H. Zinner, M.D.
All rights reserved
including the right of reproduction
in whole or in part in any form
Published by SUMMIT BOOKS
A Division of Simon & Schuster, Inc.
Simon & Schuster Building
1230 Avenue of the Americas
New York, New York 10020
SUMMIT BOOKS and colophon are trademarks of Simon & Schuster, Inc.
Manufactured in the United States of America

10   9   8   7   6   5   4   3   2   1

FIRST EDITION
Library of Congress Cataloging in Publication Data
Zinner, Stephen H., date.
    STDs—sexually transmitted diseases.
    1. Venereal diseases.   2. Hygiene, Sexual.
I. Title.   [DNLM: 1. Venereology—popular works.
WC 140 Z78s]
RC200.2.Z55   1985   616.95'1   85–2840
ISBN 0–671–49957–2

*To Meredith and Nicholas and to
the memory of Philip J. Mandelker*

Acknowledgments

About three years ago my friends Bruce Rosenzweig and Richard Rosin encouraged me to write this book. I am truly grateful for their support. I am also grateful to my friend and colleague Dr. William McCormack of Downstate Medical Center in Brooklyn, New York, for first interesting me in this topic and for serving as a valuable resource over the past fifteen years. Many thanks to Dr. Kenneth Mayer, my colleague at Brown, for his critical comments.

I am fortunate to have had excellent secretarial assistance from Jean McClain and also from Mary Ann Rao and Donna Johnson.

I am also fortunate to have worked with Kate Edgar and Jane Low, extremely careful and exacting editors.

I am grateful to my children, Meredith and Nicholas, who were so understanding while I was preoccupied with this work over the past two years.

Many thanks also to Dr. Maxim Daamen, Dr. Bernard Shepen, Dr. Joseph Levine, and Michael Groner for their social and technical support during the writing of this book.

Finally, this book would not have seen the light of day without the tireless efforts and support of my longtime and most valued friend, Jerry Wexler.

STEPHEN H. ZINNER, M.D.

Providence, Rhode Island
August 1984

Contents

9

Introduction

If the 1960s represent the years of sexual revolution, then the 1980s reflect postrevolutionary confusion, dismay, and uncertainty. Sexual activity has achieved new freedoms since the introduction of the Pill, and, with the declining use of such barrier contraceptives as the condom, epidemics of sexually transmitted diseases have erupted.

In the era of repressed sexuality that characterized much of American society during the first half of this century, venereal diseases were talked about in hushed tones and were usually thought to occur in people of low means or of less than acceptable social demeanor. It is somewhat surprising how many people are still limited in their knowledge about specific sexual practices and the correlated risk of contracting a sexually transmitted disease. This is true even among physicians and medical personnel. Medical colleagues have asked me such questions as whether one can get hepatitis by kissing or why homosexual men are so susceptible to hepatitis. Professional providers of sexual

11

pleasure, on the other hand, are sometimes more sophisticated than many physicians in matters of venereal-disease prevention. Prior to initiating sexual activity, prostitutes often feel their customer's groin for swelling of the glands, which may be symptomatic of active syphilis or other venereal diseases.

Today venereal diseases have become epidemic even in "socially acceptable" circles. Genital herpes, for example, is so prevalent among middle-class Americans that self-help groups with nationwide memberships have developed. Venereal disease no longer has quite the negative social connotations of our past, and the initials VD themselves have been replaced by STD—for "sexually transmitted disease." Even the American Venereal Disease Association has changed the name of its journal to *The Journal of Sexually Transmitted Diseases*.

If the new name for these diseases has enabled people to discuss the subject more freely, so much the better, but considerable anxiety and misinformation persist in the minds of sexually active people. It is my intention to expose some myths about sexually transmitted diseases and to relate, where possible, the specific risks or infections associated with particular sexual activities or practices.

To allay the fears and clear the confusion that surround these diseases, what is needed is a frank and open discussion of the means by which they are transmitted, the expectations for treatment and cure, and, most important, the potential for prevention of infection without having to limit sexual expression.

Many physicians in private medical settings have not been well equipped to treat patients with sexually transmitted diseases. Traditionally, medical-school curricula have given little attention to STDs, and many physicians have grown up with the concept that venereal diseases occur primarily in inner-city patients who attend city- or county-run STD clinics. Typically, medical-school lectures on sexually transmitted diseases have been highlighted with comical anecdotes that feed on the students' (and possibly the professor's) immaturity about sexuality. It is no wonder that some older physicians continue to harbor condescending attitudes toward patients with sexually transmitted diseases, their attitude being "You've had your fun, now pay for it." In the past ten years, however, younger physicians have generally become more understanding and compassionate toward STD patients, and medical-school curricula have changed in response to this widespread problem, acknowledging the importance of heightened awareness and sensitivity.

Because of the availability of federal funds, stimulated in large part by the tremendous epidemic of STDs, research in this area has increased dramatically in the past decade. Much progress has been made in understanding the dynamics, treatment, and prevention of sexually transmitted diseases, resulting from the efforts of an increasingly large number of academic physicians who have made their careers in researching these diseases. The work of these investigators has made an impact in bringing respectability to STD research.

For the most part, there is no risk of contracting a sexually transmitted disease in the absence of sexual activity. That is, these diseases are not generally transmitted by water (with a very few exceptions), towels, toilet seats, or other inanimate objects. No intimate activity is totally risk free, however, and certain sexual practices (e.g. fellatio, anal intercourse, or oral–anal contact) do increase the risk of transmission. Sex with many or multiple partners also increases this risk. Thus, it is possible to reduce the risk of transmission with minimal loss of sexual expression by *modifying* sexual activity and by being more *selective* of sexual partners. Individuals can make wiser and more appropriate choices, if they have all the facts at their disposal.

As recently as twenty years ago, a list of venereal diseases would have included only a few infections. Syphilis and gonorrhea were considered the major venereal diseases, while chancroid, lymphogranuloma venereum, and granuloma inguinale were those that occurred less frequently. Today more than eighteen disorders are known to be transmissible by various sexual practices. Some of these infections may also be transmitted by other than sexual means. For example, amebic dysentery or diarrhea caused by the *Giardia lamblia* organism may be transmitted either by oral–anal sexual contact or by water or food-borne sources.

Some of the newer sexually related diseases may themselves influence sexual behavior. The genital-herpes epidemic, which afflicts fifteen to twenty million Americans, has already produced a significant change in sexual behavior in that sexual liaisons are being scrutinized more carefully, and sexual activity has been changed or limited by many of those with this infection. Similarly, the recent development of the acquired immunodeficiency syndrome (AIDS)—although not yet proven to be related to any particular sexual practice—has frightened many homosexual men and caused them to examine and modify their own sexual practices. Ironically, that which results from sexual freedom may, in fact, limit the behavior so recently liberated.

The horizon is not so bleak, however. New drugs that do have some success against herpes viruses are available or are being developed. A newly licensed vaccine is available against hepatitis B. Research promises progress in the development of vaccines against gonorrhea, herpes, and possibly other STDs. Careful case referral and early diagnosis and treatment have reduced the spread of syphilis. There are screening clinics and services to detect the presence of nonsymptomatic gonorrheal infection and other diseases. New antibiotics are available to treat established and diagnosed infections. The presumed AIDS agent has been identified. New appreciation by physicians of the need for open, frank, and nonjudgmental treatment of homosexual patients should ease this population's access to appropriate medical care. Many sexually transmitted infections can be prevented by using such barrier methods as the condom; their increased use will most likely be associated with a dramatic decline in the incidence of these diseases.

In no way should this book substitute for a doctor's diagnosis of suspected infection. The intention of the book is not to encourage self-diagnosis but to help readers understand more fully venereal infections, especially the manifestations of early symptoms, the clinical findings and methods used by physicians to confirm diagnoses, and the recommended treatments available. Emphasis is on the known means of transmission—that is, those sexual practices that have been associated with the most likelihood of developing a given condition. Special consideration is given to known or potential preventive measures that will help the reader make the best-informed choices in terms of his or her own sexual needs.

1 / Gonorrhea

Of the sexually transmitted diseases, gonorrhea is among those with the longest recorded history. The occurrence of gonorrhea among notable poets, artists, and politicians is well documented by Theodore Rosebury in his book *Microbes and Morals*. Some of these notables include the seventeenth-century poet Thomas Carew; Samuel Johnson's biographer, James Boswell; Giovanni Casanova; Napoleon I; and probably Benito Mussolini and Adolf Hitler. Rosebury cites several references to gonorrhea in the Bible in which those with the disease are said to have the "issue." Rosebury informs us that the modern misconception about the communicability of venereal diseases by way of toilet seats may have its origins in Leviticus (15:4): "Every bed, whereon he lieth that hath the issue, is unclean: and everything, whereon he sitteth, shall be unclean."

This infection has been referred to for many years by a number of slang terms, including "the drip," "a case," "the strain," "a dose," "the bug," and "the clap," an expression probably derived from the Middle French word *clapoir*, or bordello, an assumed source of gonorrhea.

The incidence of gonorrhea among sexually active people in the last ten to fifteen years has increased astronomically, almost certainly as a result of the declining use of barrier contraceptives as well as the increased frequency of multiple sexual partners. This infection has reached epidemic proportions; more than one million cases of gonorrhea are *reported* each year.

From the beginning of the sexual revolution in the early 1960s, the number of cases of gonorrhea rose about 12 percent each year until 1978. From 1978 to 1982 the number reported decreased slightly. Occurrences of all sexually transmitted infections are thought to be grossly underreported; conservative estimates suggest that there are actually three to four million episodes of gonorrhea in the United States each year.

Gonorrhea is not age specific, but the majority of those who develop this infection are between the ages of fifteen and twenty-five. Sexually active middle-aged or elderly people, as well as infants born to women with genital gonorrhea, also contract the disease. The relatively uncommon form that afflicts infants is gonococcal conjunctivitis. In most countries, however, the routine use of preventive eyedrops has dramatically decreased its occurrence. Gonorrhea rarely infects the fetus during pregnancy. If this occurs, however, the baby may be delivered prematurely or may develop arthritis or systemic gonococcal infection.

The organism responsible for gonorrhea is the gonococcus. Discovered in 1879 by the microbiologist Albert

Neisser, the bacterium is known formally as *Neisseria gonorrhoeae*. The disease-causing strains of the gonococcus can adhere to the mucous membranes that line the back of the mouth and throat, the rectum, the urethra, and the endocervix. Most skin, including that of the penis and the walls of the vagina, are lined with a different kind of epithelial cell to which the gonococcus cannot adhere. Thus, gonorrhea is rarely transmitted by nongenital contact.

When the gonorrheal bacteria stick to the surface cells, they begin to set up housekeeping and multiply. When these organisms multiply, they then invade the tissues between the cells and produce an irritating substance that causes inflammation. This inflammation brings white blood cells to the site of invasion, causing many of the characteristic symptoms of gonorrhea.

Gonorrheal infection is usually transmitted by vaginal intercourse, anal intercourse, or oral sex. That is, it is transmitted by direct contact between the mucous membranes lining the opening of the penis (the urethral orifice), the uterine cervix, the back of the throat, or the rectum with infected material which may also come from any of these sites. Gonorrhea is not likely to be transmitted by sharing a drink or by intimate kissing. Gonorrhea of the urethra can develop as the result of oral sex with a man or woman with gonococcal infection of the throat, but this occurs less frequently than developing gonorrhea of the throat as a result of oral sex. Saliva cannot kill the gonococcus. Women can develop anal or rectal gonorrhea without having had anal intercourse, because vaginal discharges containing the bacteria can be transmitted from the vagina to the rectum by fingers or penis without direct penetration. As mentioned, gonorrhea may be transmitted to the eyes of newborns as they come into contact with the bacteria while passing through the birth canal. Gonococcal conjunctivitis may also be spread to adults or children if infected material from the genitals is transferred to the eyes by way of the fingers.

Not every contact with the gonococcus results in infection. Only about 50 percent of women whose sexual partners have gonorrhea will in fact become infected. For a man whose sexual partner has gonorrhea, the risk of infection may be as low as 20 to 30 percent.

The risk of developing gonorrhea increases with homosexual men, primarily because the asymptomatic nature of gonorrhea of the throat or rectum allows transmission to occur unknowingly. The risk of gonorrhea also increases with higher numbers of sexual partners, and the frequency of anonymous sexual contacts makes control of this infection difficult.

Many other STDs may occur simultaneously with gonorrhea. It is not uncommon for people with gonorrhea to develop symptoms of this infection while also incubating another sexually transmitted disease such as syphilis. Similarly, *Chlamydia trachomatis*, one of the organisms responsible for nongonococcal urethritis, may also be present simultaneously with the gonococcus. Most of the treatment regimens available for gonorrhea also cure syphilis in the incubating stages. However, not all of the treatment regimens for gonorrhea are effective against chlamydial infections (see Chapter 3).

SYMPTOMS

Gonorrhea may or may not cause symptoms, but an asymptomatic infection is just as contagious and potentially serious a disease as a symptomatic one. The primary symptoms of gonorrhea in men are pain and burning on urination and the presence of an involuntary drip from the urethra at the tip of the penis. This puslike material is yellow and thick and may be sticky. Most men who develop symptomatic gonorrhea after infection will develop these symptoms within two to ten days after contact with an infected partner. However, men with gonorrheal infection may remain without symptoms for a longer time. (In one study, more than 60 percent of men with gonorrhea were found to be asymptomatic.) It is obvious that these men are at great risk of unknowingly transmitting their disease to sexual contacts.

Men and women, whether homosexual or heterosexual, who practice oral-genital sex or rectal intercourse may have gonorrhea of the rectum or throat with no obvious symptoms. However, some people may experience itching or a discharge around the anus, and those with gonorrhea of the throat may develop a sore throat. About 5 percent of women and 25 percent of homosexual men attending STD clinics have gonorrhea of the throat as evidenced by gonococcal cultures. Up to 40 percent of women with cervical gonorrhea may also have rectal infections (often without symptoms).

In women, the classic symptom of gonorrhea is pelvic inflammatory disease, or PID (inflammation of the fallopian tubes). It usually causes severe lower-abdominal or pelvic pain and is often accompanied by an unpleasant-smelling vaginal discharge. Women with pus in the fallopian tubes may develop high fevers and be quite ill. PID may be present in 50 percent or more of women with any symptoms related to gonorrhea. (Many other organisms, however, may also cause this syndrome.) PID may cause impaired fertility and may be associated with an increased risk of ectopic pregnancy.

Many women report only nonspecific symptoms of gonorrhea, which include common complaints of malaise and not feeling right. More specific symptoms may develop within two weeks or longer following exposure to an infected sexual partner. Some women with gonorrheal infection develop small abscesses in the glands around the vagina. Others develop symptoms similar to those produced by urinary infections, such as increased frequency of urination or pain, burning, or difficulty on urination. Sometimes a puslike discharge is the only symptom present.

Some say as many as 80 percent of women with gonorrhea have no specific symptoms. This figure, however, may be exaggerated, since it is derived only from examinations of women referred to STD clinics as a result of being exposed to gonorrhea. These female contacts may or may not have had time to develop symptoms.

In about 1 percent of both sexes, untreated gonorrhea may become widespread in the bloodstream, in addition to manifesting itself through local symptoms. In the bloodstream, gonorrhea may produce fever, swelling of the joints, arthritis, or widely spread lesions on the skin which may look like small blisters on a red base. This disseminated gonorrheal infection may occur during pregnancy or around the time of the menstrual period. It may develop in people with asymptomatic gonorrhea at any site.

In the days before the development of effective antibiotic treatment for gonorrhea, serious consequences occurred. Men and (rarely) women who developed stricture of the urinary passage required dilation (stretching) treatments by urologic specialists. Women with pelvic inflammatory disease often became sterile as a result of chronic and repeated infections. On rare occasions serious or fatal infections of the nervous system or heart also occurred, as well as meningitis. These complications rarely occur today with prompt treatment.

DIAGNOSIS

Diagnosis of gonorrhea must be made on the basis of a laboratory examination of a specimen from an infected site. Many people harbor the misconception that if their premarital blood test or blood test for VD is negative, they couldn't possibly have gonorrhea. This is not the case. These blood tests simply detect antibodies produced by a past or present infection with *syphilis*. Although a great deal of research under way suggests that it may soon be possible to detect certain antibodies to the gonococcus, these tests are not yet fully developed.

In diagnosing men with genital gonorrhea, a physician usually obtains a sample of the discharge (the drip) to make a smear on a glass slide which is stained and then examined under a high-powered microscope. The presence of inflammatory cells (white blood cells or pus) packed with the organism of gonorrhea (the gonococcus) will confirm the diagnosis.

A slide smear, however, is not always accurate in detecting gonorrhea in asymptomatic men who have had sexual contacts with others known to have gonorrhea or in men who are at risk of contracting gonorrhea of the throat or rectum. In these cases, samples of the suspected infected material are taken from the penis, the throat, and the rectum with a swab and then cultured in a bacteriology laboratory. Slide smears made from the throat and the rectum are not useful in making a positive diagnosis because the normal organisms present in these sites can sometimes mimic the gonococcus or be present in such large numbers as to obscure the presence of gonococcal organisms on the smear. A culture, however, allows for the isolation and ultimate identification of these organisms from any suspected site. Results from a culture usually take forty-eight hours.

To confirm the diagnosis, it is strongly advised that in *all* cases of gonorrhea a culture be obtained, as well as a smear. This is especially important if gonorrhea is suspected in spite of negative test results of a slide smear.

In diagnosing women with symptomatic or asymptomatic gonorrhea of the cervix, a physician usually obtains a culture of the material taken from the cervical opening, although a fairly reliable diagnosis can be made on the basis of a stained smear in symptomatic women with genital gonorrhea. Results from a smear can be obtained in a few minutes as opposed to a culture, which requires several days for the organisms to be identified. Urine cultures may also reveal the gonococcus. Obtaining a culture is the most reliable way of confirming the presence of gonorrhea, whether or not symptoms are present.

No medical test is perfect. Occasionally even cultures from presumed infected sites may not yield positive results when, in fact, the gonococcus is present. Repeated cultures may be necessary. In well over 90 percent of the cases, however, a doctor can be reasonably certain whether the infection is present based on a culture.

The development of new immunologic techniques and the use of highly specific monoclonal antibodies are likely to revolutionize the diagnosis of gonorrhea and other STDs. Undoubtedly they will make possible the prompt identification of the gonococcus in direct smears from the urethra or the cervix, as well as the pharynx (throat) or the rectum. A high degree of accuracy will be achieved with the use of these new techniques. Although none of these rapid tests are in current widespread use, most will likely become available within the next few years.

TREATMENT

Fortunately, gonorrhea is not only treatable but also almost always curable. A wide variety of effective antibiotics are available. Penicillin and its relatives, ampicillin and amoxicillin, are the major drugs used in the treatment of gonorrhea. However, many people have expressed the fear that penicillin will no longer be active against gonorrhea organisms because they have steadily become more resistant to penicillin. Larger doses of penicillin are now required to cure most strains of the gonococcus.

Of greater concern is the increasing number of people

infected with strains of the gonococcus that are totally resistant to penicillin. Fortunately, such antibiotics as spectinomycin and tetracycline are effective in curing these infections and can also be used by those who have an allergy to penicillin.

Depending on the type of infection, various antibiotics may be prescribed either in single doses or in doses taken over a period of several days. Sometimes antibiotics are used together with another drug that delays excretion by the kidney and thus maintains higher levels of the antibiotic in the blood and the tissue. Similarly, two doses of penicillin taken intramuscularly, combined with the oral administration of an excretion-blocking drug, are also effective. Tetracycline must be taken two to four times a day for a week. Treatment with any antibiotic should be continued for the entire prescribed course even after symptoms have disappeared. Incomplete treatment may lead to recurrence or may contribute to the emergence of resistant organisms.

Treatment of pharyngeal and rectal gonorrhea requires special attention by a physician because eradication of the gonococcus from these sites is more difficult. These infections are curable, however.

New drugs that are effective against gonorrhea are being produced and released for use in the United States at a rapid rate. Some of these new drugs are already being used by physicians.

While being treated for gonorrhea, you should refrain from all sexual activity until your doctor can determine that you are no longer infected. This requires a posttreatment culture four to seven days following treatment, and it takes about forty-eight hours to complete the test. Remember that a single episode of gonorrhea at any site does not prevent subsequent infection at the same or a different site as a result of reexposure.

Pregnant women with gonorrhea can also be treated with antibiotics. A woman undergoing evaluation for gonorrhea or any STD should always tell her doctor if she is pregnant.

PREVENTION

Unfortunately, there is currently no vaccine for the prevention of gonorrhea, although current research may soon lead to the development of such a vaccine. One episode of gonorrhea will not prevent subsequent attacks, which may be due to different strains of the organism or to the individual's lack of immunity to the same strain. Immunity is not induced in the same manner as in the case of chicken pox or measles, for instance. The details of resistance to gonorrheal infection are not yet well known.

The use of single doses of such antibiotics as penicillin and tetracycline immediately following sexual contact with an infected person may reduce the risk of developing infection. However, the danger inherent in this preventive approach is that the infecting organisms will become increasingly resistant to whatever antibiotic is used.

Using a condom will prevent the transmission of gonorrhea from the penis to another susceptible area. Indeed, the risk and incidence of gonorrhea would be reduced dramatically if condoms were used regularly. Obviously, the condom must fit properly and be completely intact.

Any small tear, puncture, or hole in the condom will allow for the transmission of the gonococcus. Although careful washing of the genital area with soap and water can reduce the number of potential infecting organisms present, cleanliness is not adequate in itself to prevent transmission of gonorrhea. Using a diaphragm will not prevent cervical gonococcal infection, but some spermicidal creams, foams, and jellies do have some success against the organism. They do not reliably prevent gonorrhea, however.

Since gonorrhea often produces no symptoms (or produces nonspecific symptoms), routine screening for the gonococcus will identify infection and indicate the need for treatment to eradicate the infection and prevent unwitting spread to sexual partners. People who are sexually active with many partners should be cultured about four times a year.

By law, all cases of gonorrhea must be reported to the health department. This is generally done by your doctor or by the laboratory identifying the organism. This information is used in strict confidence to help you identify and notify your recent sexual partners (within two to four weeks) whom you might have infected or from whom you contracted the infection. These records are not made available to any public or private source. Only by careful and confidential contact tracing can all infected partners be identified early enough and then treated to limit further spread of the disease. If treatment is begun early, gonorrhea usually leaves no serious complications. Because of the asymptomatic nature of this infection, it is often difficult to be certain who actually infected you.

2 / Genital Herpes

No common sexually transmitted disease has captured the headlines and threatened to change the sexual habits of modern Americans more than genital herpes. Although this disease was known in the eighteenth and nineteenth centuries, it was the sexual revolution of the 1970s that brought genital herpes into worldwide prominence.

Up until the early part of this century, this condition was believed to be due to various toxins or irritants and was often seen in patients who had other sexually transmitted diseases, namely gonorrhea and syphilis. As recently as ten to fifteen years ago, it was not uncommon for physicians to identify sores and lesions as resulting from toxins and irritants rather than herpes. It is interesting, however, that the descriptions in early textbooks of venereal disease clearly describe not only the appearance of these lesions but the now well-known tendency for them to recur at identical sites under periods of stress and illness, as well as spontaneously.

Associated with the widespread use of the Pill and with the liberalization of sexual practices, genital herpes has become more prevalent, along with the other sexually transmitted diseases. The number of consultations with physicians and other health-care providers for genital herpes has steadily increased during the past ten to fifteen years. It is likely that these numbers have increased approximately 10 percent every year.

Herpes is a disease caused by a virus. This virus is related to, but differs from, viruses that cause infectious mononucleosis, chicken pox, and shingles. Unlike bacteria, viruses cannot be seen with an ordinary light microscope, nor can they be grown in artificial media or culture plates. Viruses can be grown, however, in tissue cultures available in specialized laboratories. Viruses are intracellular pathogens, and, as such, they require cells in which to grow. In the laboratory, these cells are provided in tissues grown in culture. The presence of the virus can be identified by characteristic damage to these cells.

Herpes simplex virus (HSV, the virus that causes both genital herpes and cold sores) can be cultured from the lesions up to seven to ten days after they appear (longer after the first attack). Although tissue cultures are not available routinely, more laboratories are becoming available to the physician for use in isolating the herpes organism.

The herpes virus consists of a DNA core plus a protein coat. In order for herpes virus and other viruses to produce disease, they must inhabit a living cell. Once the virus has gained access to a cell it is incorporated into the cell's machinery: the cell's own protein factory begins to make copies of the infecting virus, which can then leave and infect other cells, repeating the cycle.

Once a person gets HSV, protective mechanisms in the body help minimize widespread infection either by preventing replication of the virus or by neutralizing the virus to prevent it from attaching to or entering an uninfected cell. Interferon, for example, is a substance that is secreted by virus-infected cells to prevent simultaneous infection by a second or different type of virus. As a result, interferon and other protective mechanisms generally limit the spread of herpes virus infections to a few body sites. In patients with normal host defenses (and this includes almost all patients who develop genital herpes) the infection is contained to a limited area of the body. It is very unusual for widespread infection of herpes to occur except in newborns, who do not have well-developed immune systems, and in people with underlying diseases that affect immunity in general.

During the phase of intracellular herpes virus multiplication, damage to a given tissue area is usually due to destruction of the infected cell with the release of irritating and/or toxic products. This results in the local lesions or symptoms of the herpes infection. Unlike bacteria, which produce pus or inflammation as in gonorrhea, herpes virus produces well-localized lesions, or sores, usually at the primary site of infection.

Herpes simplex virus and the related virus of chicken pox and shingles (Varicella-Zoster virus) also have the ability to remain latent for a lifetime. In the case of genital herpes, it is thought that the organism first gains access to a nerve ending serving the area of primary infection and then travels to the root of this nerve, where it may remain latent.

This concept of latency is poorly understood but is most likely responsible for the tendency of herpes infections to recur at the same site or near the same physical area.

This latency phenomenon has made it difficult to cure or eradicate herpes infection. Most antiviral drugs are not effective against the virus in its latent state. What activates a virus from its latent to its infectious state is not completely understood, but such events as menstruation, stress, trauma, irritation, other serious bacterial infections and illnesses, sunlight exposure, and emotional distress have all been thought to be responsible.

There are two subtypes of herpes simplex viruses that cause infections in humans. These virus subtypes are only slightly different in some of the chemical components of their outer coat. Typically, herpes simplex virus Type 1 (HSV-1) has been associated with herpes of the mouth and the lips. Herpes simplex virus Type 2 (HSV-2) has typically been associated with genital herpes infections. However, with changing sexual practices both of these viruses can be found in lesions at both sites.

Oral herpes infection (HSV-1) manifests as recurrent cold sores around the lips and mouth, whereas genital herpes (HSV-2) manifests as similar recurrent lesions about the genitalia. People with oral herpes (HSV-1) during its active state may transmit this infection to the genitalia of their sexual partners during oral sex, and those with genital herpes (HSV-2) similarly may transmit HSV-2 to the oral area.

Unfortunately, details of the actual transmission of HSV-2 during sexual activity are not known. It is clear, however, that the virus can be transmitted through oral–

genital, genital–genital, or genital–anal contact. Studies on the risk of transmissibility (that is, what percentage of susceptible individuals that have sexual contact with people with genital-herpes lesions will in fact develop the lesions themselves) are in progress now. It is unlikely that herpes is spread by nonintimate contact or by the use of hot tubs or shared towels.

Prior to the sexual revolution, most healthy adults could be found to have antibodies in their blood serum that were directed primarily against HSV-1. The presence of antibodies to a given virus reflects past exposure to the agent without the person's necessarily having had detectable lesions. These antibodies may protect against, or modify, the expression of genital herpes. Today the proportion of normal young adults with antibodies to HSV-1 is somewhat lower, around 50 to 60 percent; the reason for this change is unclear. However, antibodies to both HSV-1 and HSV-2 are quite common in people who are close contacts of those with known genital herpes infections. The presence or absence of these antibodies may influence the severity of herpes infections.

Manifestations of genital-herpes infection differ depending on the presence of HSV-1 antibodies in the blood. Most studies of genital herpes describe two types of initial genital infection: (1) the *primary* infection with either the HSV-1 or HSV-2 virus, and (2) the *nonprimary* infection, that is, the initial manifestation of genital infection in a person who already has the HSV-1 serum antibody, implying previous experience with one of the herpes viruses (HSV-1), with no detectable lesions. Both of these initial infections are more severe than are recurrent episodes of genital herpes, with primary infections being the most severe. However, genital lesions due to HSV-1 (up to 30 percent of cases) may be less severe and recur less frequently than infections due to HSV-2.

About 60 to 70 percent of patients may experience one or more recurrent attacks. (The major concern of people with herpes is this recurrence and the consequent limitations put on sexual activity. In many cases the psychological implications of genital herpes infection may be worse than the actual disease itself.) The frequency of recurrent episodes is not clearly known, but frequent recurrences do not necessarily imply the presence of any abnormality in the immune system. (On the other hand, patients who do have known underlying immune disorders may be subject to serious infection with herpes simplex virus.) In time, the number of recurrences per year begins to decrease, and eventually many patients report the disease less frequently. The recurrences may disappear completely or "burn out" after several years. Some patients (up to 30 or 40 percent) never experience a recurrent attack.

Rarely, some people may spread herpes to sexual contacts without knowledge of ever having had the infection. Many people with primary infection will shed virus for up to eleven or more days. Most people will stop shedding the virus within three weeks of the onset of infection, and in people with nonprimary herpes (those with the serum antibody to HSV-1) the virus may be shed for a shorter period. In recurrent genital-herpes lesions, viral shedding is even shorter, and most people will stop shedding by five days, although this may continue up to ten to eleven days. There is very little shedding of viruses during the interval between recurrent attacks (less than 5 percent in women). Shedding refers to the presence of culturable virus at a site. This suggests that the risk of transmitting genital-herpes infection by means of sexual intercourse when lesions are not present in the genitalia must be very low.

The type of person who becomes infected with genital herpes is difficult to define in detail, primarily because national reporting for this disease is not required. However, it is clear that genital-herpes infection is not limited to patients who seek care in inner-city STD clinics. It appears that most patients with this disease are Caucasians between the ages of twenty and forty and earn more than twenty thousand dollars per year. Although gonorrhea is prevalent among homosexually active men, genital herpes is ten times *less* frequent in this population than is gonorrhea. (Homosexual men are subject to developing anal infection with herpes simplex virus, however.) Most people who go to private physicians to be treated for genital herpes are heterosexually active.

Herpes in pregnancy is of special concern. Genital herpes in a pregnant woman may result in infection of the newborn, and the known presence of active herpes infection is likely to result in delivery by cesarean section to prevent neonatal herpes infection. The risk to the fetus is greatest during a primary infection and less during recurrent attacks. If the fetus is infected during pregnancy (in utero) there may be an early fetal death (stillbirth). Most cases of fetal infection are caused by direct spreading of the virus to the intrauterine contents during rupture of the membranes or during delivery, although infection may also be caused by cross-placental spreading from the mother's bloodstream. Stillbirths, spontaneous abortion, congenital anomalies, or early delivery may occur. Pregnant women with a history of genital herpes are often studied or cultured for herpes at frequent intervals near term. These tests or cultures are more reliable than the absence of symptoms or lesions. Vaginal delivery is usually safe if there is no evidence of active viral shedding or herpetic lesions.

Neonatal infection may result in local infection with vesicles on the skin or in the eye or the mouth. Meningitis, encephalitis, or disseminated herpes infection may occur. Treatment with vidarabine or acyclovir may reduce the high mortality rate of disseminated infection. Local infections may tend to recur but can generally be treated.

SYMPTOMS

The first signs of genital herpes infection may begin two to ten days or longer after exposure to a person with either genital-herpes lesions or virus shed from a nonsymptomatic genital site. There are often, but not always, a few early, prelesion symptoms which may include a tingling sensation, a dull ache or pain, or an itching sensation in the genital area. This is followed by the appearance of tiny pimples (also known as vesicles) that initially are clear but may soon become cloudy and pustular. These clustered lesions are small and may be no more than one or two millimeters in diameter.

In men the primary lesions occur most frequently on the shaft of the penis, but they may also occur around the anus, in the skin of the pubic area, or even along the thigh. In women the early lesions may occur around the lips of the vagina (both the labia majora and the labia minora), or they may occur near the clitoris, urethra, buttock, anus, pubic area, or on the thigh. In the initial attack the lesions last approximately five to six days, during which time the vesicles become unroofed, and small, shallow, painful, moist ulcers appear and may last as long as six to eight days before they begin to crust, roughly two weeks after the initial appearance. By three weeks after onset most patients no longer have symptoms of this infection, although some sensation of the sores may persist longer.

Primary HSV-2 genital infection tends to be more severe in women than in men. Women may complain of severe vaginal itching and pain as well as extremely painful intercourse. Nonprimary initial infections in people who have the serum antibody to HSV-1 may have fewer complications than in those people who lack such an antibody. In the initial true primary infection (serum antibodies lacking), fever, malaise, swollen lymph nodes in the groin, painful urination, headache, and other symptoms may occur. Primary infections in women are more likely to be associated with symptoms of urethritis, constitutional symptoms including fever, malaise, and headache, and extragenital lesions (for example, those on the buttock, the groin, or the fingers). In addition, primary lesions in women may take longer to heal than those in men.

Other complications of initial genital-herpes infection include retention of urine (possibly requiring catheterization), infection with herpes of the finger, the rectum, or the uterus, and very rarely meningitis. None of these complications is very common.

Although herpes can recur at the genital locations, there

are no long-term side effects on fertility, sexual potency, or general health. The association between genital-herpes infection and the occurrence of cervical cancer has been well publicized. The evidence is not conclusive but is of concern. Yearly Pap smears are therefore recommended for women with herpes.

Recurrent episodes of genital-herpes infection in general are much milder than the initial attack in both men and women; and in women, recurrent lesions are almost always limited to the external genitalia. As in the initial infection, there may be prelesion symptoms of itching, burning, or tingling at previous infection sites. The same pimplelike lesions occur, but these usually heal completely within six to eight days or earlier. The degree of pain may be less than at the time of the primary infection, and in most people the pain disappears within a week. Recurrent infections appear to be somewhat more severe in women than in men (as with primary infections), and the presence of systemic symptoms and pain and burning on urination, as well as the duration of pain in the herpes lesions, are also greater in women than in men.

DIAGNOSIS

The diagnosis of genital herpes is usually made by inspection of the lesions and by a smear prepared from a sample scraped from the base of one of these lesions. The smear does not reveal the virus itself, but reveals the presence of certain cellular features that suggest infection with herpes virus. Proof of this diagnosis is made by culturing the virus in a viral laboratory. Other new rapid slide identification tests are now available for routine use. These tests use a flourescent-labeled highly specific antibody to detect the presence of herpes virus in the smears.

Other sexually transmitted diseases, including syphilis, chancroid, donovanosis (granuloma inguinale), lymphogranuloma venereum, traumatic genital ulcers, yeast infections, and drug reactions, can mimic genital-herpes infection to some degree. Some patients with genital ulcers may have more than one of the above causes responsible for their lesion. Blood tests are not helpful in the specific diagnosis of genital herpes, but blood tests for the presence of antibodies to HSV-2 may be useful in establishing recent or past herpes infection.

TREATMENT

Until very recently there has been no effective therapy for any form of genital-herpes infection. Numerous possible treatments have been advocated from a variety of sources, and these have often led to false hopes for sufferers from this disease. A number of drugs have been studied but have been found to be ineffective. These include 2-deoxy-D-glucose, idoxuridine, adenine arabinoside (Vira-A), iodine, zinc, lysine, thymol, and ether. All of these have been tried topically and have not been proved effective in controlled-treatment trials. Some of the proposed treatments, in fact, have potentially serious side effects and are ineffective against herpes. In general, smallpox and tuberculosis vaccinations, meant to stimulate the immune response, have also been unsuccessful.

Topical and oral therapy are the most practical methods

of treatment and have the most widespread use for people with first attacks of genital-herpes infection. For example, the recently introduced drug acyclovir (Zovirax) has been proved to reduce the shedding of virus, shorten the duration of symptoms, and facilitate the complete healing of lesions when topically applied or when given orally. In very severe cases of genital-herpes infection, some physicians may even recommend intravenous therapy with acyclovir.

At the present time, there is very little hard evidence to suggest that topical acyclovir treatment can prolong the duration of symptom-free intervals between attacks and reduce the frequency of recurrence. Low-dose continuous treatment with oral acyclovir is useful in reducing the frequency of recurrence, and is used in people with severe, closely spaced recurrences. It is unlikely, however, that acyclovir in any form will be useful as a cure for herpes simplex. The drug can neither affect the latent virus at the nerve root cell nor prevent the virus from reaching the nerve root.

Other drugs are currently being tested. It is possible that the genetically engineered production of interferon in bacterial cells may be useful in the treatment of this disease, at least with respect to decreasing recurrent episodes. People with recurrent infections may find some relief from warm soaks or sitz baths and also from the application of a topical anesthetic agent such as viscous Xylocaine.

Many people suffering from herpes infection are seriously troubled emotionally by the presence of their disease. In addition to many local groups, a nationally organized support group, the Herpes Resource Center, formerly known as Herpetics Engaged in Living Productively (HELP), is available to provide information and general support to sufferers from this disease. It can be reached in care of the American Social Health Association, P.O. Box 100, Palo Alto, CA 94302. This herpes resource center also publishes a newsletter for its members which contains up-to-the-minute useful information. Membership in the center costs twenty dollars.

PREVENTION

The use of a well-fitted condom will offer some degree of protection from herpes infection, but only in those areas that are covered by the condom. For example, if during sexual intercourse the skin around the genitalia has active herpetic lesions, then skin-to-skin contact (unprotected by the condom) will allow potential transmission of this agent. The use of a diaphragm will not prevent spread of this infection. As with many other STDs, it is likely that limiting the number of sexual partners will certainly decrease the risk of acquiring genital-herpes infection. Even those with recurrent genital herpes may be reinfected with new strains of the virus from a partner with another type of active herpes virus infection. Also, herpes can be spread from a genital site to another part of the body. Careful hand-washing after touching the genitals will reduce this risk.

A major problem, as yet unsolved, is the fact that viral shedding may begin prior to the onset of symptoms or the appearance of obvious lesions. Minimal symptoms may be ignored, and the virus may be present prior to the eruption of a sore. Therefore sexual intercourse should not take place if any of these symptoms are present, however minimal.

Although the development of any useful vaccine is still in progress, two approaches have been suggested. One of the vaccines under current study is likely to be effective in modifying the symptoms and eruption associated with recurrent infection. Another vaccine under consideration, directed at reducing the rate of infection and thereby preventing the induction of the latent state, has been tested recently and appears to be promising. There is no known effective cure for herpes, and its ability to remain in a latent form within a nerve root cell may militate against an ultimate cure by an antiviral drug.

Sexual activity should be avoided during an attack of genital herpes. Few people so infected, however, will want to engage in sex, because of the painful lesions.

Pregnant women with primary or recurrent genital herpes must inform their physician or other health-care provider of their pregnancy. Careful monitoring at the time of delivery will help minimize infection of the newborn.

It is often difficult to be certain which sexual partner may have spread this infection. It's important, therefore, to inform recent sexual partners (within the last four weeks) of their possible exposure to herpes so that they can seek treatment. Physicians are not legally required to report herpes to the health department.

3 / Chlamydia Infections and Nongonococcal Urethritis in Men

Early after the identification of the gonococcus as the cause of classical gonorrhea, physicians began using the terms "specific urethritis" to refer to gonorrhea in men, and "nonspecific urethritis," or "nongonococcal urethritis," to refer to a condition in men with similar symptoms but in which the gonococcal organism could not be found. Specific and nonspecific urethritis also occur in women, but these are commonly referred to as urinary-tract infections rather than urethritis, since they produce similar symptoms and may involve other urinary structures in addition to the urethra itself. For a discussion of urinary-tract and chlamydia infections in women, see Chapters 4 and 5.

In the last century and up until the modern microbiological era, physicians felt that nongonococcal urethritis in men resulted from a variety of causes. For example, it was widely thought that sexual intercourse with a woman during, or shortly after, menstruation resulted in the development of urethritis due to some product of "putrefaction" of the menstrual flow. Other presumed causes included frequent or heavy sexual intercourse, the placing of foreign objects in the urethra, sex with an "unclean" woman, frequent masturbation, and sodomy.

Today nongonococcal urethritis is the sexually transmitted disease that probably causes more visits to venereal-disease clinics or private physicians than any other. Unlike gonorrhea or syphilis, nongonococcal urethritis does not have to be reported by a physician to the health department; therefore, estimates of its occurrence are inaccurate at best. Nonetheless, nongonococcal urethritis (NGU) is frequent in sexually active men and is probably 50 to 100 percent more common than gonorrhea. This disease is especially frequent in white middle-class men and is alleged to be more frequent than gonorrhea in men who are circumcised.

One form of NGU, postgonococcal urethritis, manifests as a thin watery urethral discharge from the penis roughly one to two weeks after successful treatment of true gonorrhea with penicillin. It is probably due to the simultaneous infection with the gonococcus and one of the organisms that are now known to produce nongonococcal urethritis. Since penicillin is effective treatment for gonorrhea but not for NGU, the similar, but not identical, symptoms of NGU may become apparent only after the gonorrhea is treated.

It is only within the last ten years that the causative organisms have been identified for most cases of nongonococcal urethritis in men. About one half of all cases are due to the organism known as *Chlamydia trachomatis*. The *Chlamydia trachomatis* organism may also be present in the opening of the uterus in about 5 to 20 percent of healthy asymptomatic women, and in 25 to 45 percent of women who have had sexual contacts with men having NGU (see Chapter 4). Since the organisms may be present without symptoms in the cervix of women, the development of this infection in a man does not necessarily imply sexual infidelity. It is the same organism (or a very similar strain thereof) that causes trachoma, a leading cause of blindness in the world, though this form of blindness is not sexually transmitted and is not associated with nongonococcal urethritis. (Nor is trachoma common in the United States or Western Europe.) In addition, one strain of *Chlamydia trachomatis* is now known to cause the disease lymphogranuloma venereum (see Chapter 10).

The presence of the chlamydia organism associated with sexually transmitted diseases is also known to be responsible for congenital conjunctivitis and pneumonia in newborns of mothers who have this organism present in their genital tract at the time of delivery. The chlamydia organism also can cause pelvic inflammatory disease (PID) and is probably second only to the gonococcus as a cause of this syndrome in women (see Chapter 4).

Ureaplasma urealyticum (which is known as one of the genital mycoplasmas) has been recognized as another cause of nongonococcal urethritis. This organism has been demonstrated to be present in the urethra of men and in the vagina of women who do not have any specific symptoms. This organism, however, is usually found only in sexually active people; its presence is much less frequent in men and women with few lifetime sexual partners. The *Trichomonas vaginalis* parasite can cause urethritis or prostatitis in men (and it often causes vaginitis and cervicitis in women—see Chapter 4). Other known (such as yeasts, wart virus, and herpes simplex virus) or as yet unidentified organisms are responsible for the remaining cases of NGU in sexually active men.

SYMPTOMS

The classic symptom of NGU is a urethral drip that is different from that of gonorrhea. Whereas gonorrhea typically produces a thick, yellow, puslike discharge, the discharge of nongonococcal urethritis is thinner and less copious. It is typically described as mucoid and is probably the same discharge that was known as gleet in the early part of this century. Some men, however, may not develop this symptom at all. The incubation period of nongonococcal urethritis is considerably longer than that of gonorrhea and may take up to two to three weeks following exposure. These organisms may persist for many years in healthy women, and although they may produce some cervical erosions, they may not be associated with distinct symptoms that would cause women to seek diagnosis and treatment. For this reason, both partners should be examined and treated when NGU is suspected, to prevent reinfection.

Nongonococcal urethritis is associated with penile itching and some burning on urination but to a lesser degree than that associated with gonorrhea. The *Chlamydia trachomatis* organism of NGU may also produce in men a swelling of the epididymis (the tubules leading from the testes to the urethra). This occurs as swelling and tenderness near the testicle and may also be associated with fever.

The symptoms of NGU may wax and wane and may recur frequently even after appropriate treatment. A thin watery discharge may last for several months, spontaneously disappear without treatment, and again recur with or without treatment. The organisms of NGU are more unpredictable than the gonococcus, but usually there are no long-term local or systemic consequences of nongonococcal urethritis. However, some men with NGU do de-develop epididymitis (see Chapter 10), mild to moderately severe arthritis, skin rash, conjunctivitis, or other eye problems. This symptom complex is known as Reiter's syndrome and is associated with chlamydial urethral infection. It may be quite debilitating but usually can be treated with various forms of antiinflammatory drugs. Epididymitis or prostatitis may sometimes result as a complication of NGU, but prompt treatment will usually prevent this. There is no evidence that NGU can produce male infertility.

Homosexual men who practice anal intercourse are at risk of transmitting this chlamydial disease from the penis to the rectum, resulting in proctitis (see Chapter 8), or from the rectum to the penis. In the rectum the strain of chlamydia associated with lymphogranuloma venereum may cause irritation and inflammation of the anus and rectum which may result in painful defecation with or without mucus and blood.

It is important to recognize that more than one type of organism may be responsible for discharge from the penis. The organisms may be associated with gonorrhea or nongonococcal urethritis, and both may be present simultaneously.

DIAGNOSIS

The diagnosis of NGU is made by examination of the discharge. The absence of any stainable bacteria looking like gonococci is highly suggestive of nongonococcal urethritis. When there is no discharge but other NGU symptoms are present, the physician may insert a thin swab into the urethra to make a smear. Alternatively, a sample of first voided urine can be spun in a centrifuge and smeared on a slide. These smears are examined for the presence of inflammatory white blood cells without bacteria. A culture should also be obtained to rule out the presence of gonorrhea.

The culture identifying the organisms often responsible for nongonococcal urethritis, *Chlamydia trachomatis* or *Ureaplasma urealyticum*, is not routinely available in all hospitals or clinic laboratories but may become more available over the next few years. A new slide fluorescent antibody test is available for the rapid identification of chlamydia in the discharge, and another method, which utilizes an enzyme immunoassay, is also available. The culture of these organisms is not absolutely necessary for diagnosing nongonococcal urethritis in men. A relatively reliable diagnosis can be based on a history, a physical exam, and a slide smear.

In men with nongonococcal urethritis it is also important to rule out the presence of the small parasite *Trichomonas vaginalis*. This organism is identified on examination and culture of a drop of fresh urine for men and a drop of vaginal fluid for women. *Trichomonas* may cause symptomatic or nonsymptomatic urethritis in men who have sexual intercourse with an infected woman. The symptoms include penile itching, painful urination, and a small amount of discharge.

TREATMENT

Several antibiotics, including tetracycline and erythromycin, are effective against NGU organisms. A form of tetracycline is prescribed most usually, and the treatment generally continues for ten days. Some of these organisms are also sensitive to sulfa drugs and spectinomycin.

Nonsymptomatic sexual partners of men with chlamydial urethritis should also be treated. Similarly, men who have intercourse with a woman known to have chlamydial cervical or pelvic infection should be treated. This treatment of both sexual partners will prevent reinfection and reduce the frequency of recurrent chlamydial infections in sexually active people.

Trichomoniasis can be treated easily with the oral drug metronidazole (Flagyl). Steady sexual partners of men with trichomonal urethritis should also be treated even in the absence of symptoms, to help minimize or prevent recurrent episodes in either partner.

PREVENTION

Prevention of nongonococcal urethritis is probably limited to condom use only. If organisms are present in a woman's vagina or on the cervix, the condom will prevent exposure of the male urethra to these organisms. Similarly, in men with nongonococcal urethritis condom use will prevent transmission of the organisms to an uninfected partner. The use of a diaphragm does not provide protection from these infections.

General hygienic measures such as washing of the genitalia and douching may reduce somewhat the risk of infection, although this has not been proved. Indeed, overzealous douching in women can lead to vaginal irritation and result in increased susceptibility to infection.

Treatment of sexual partners of both men and women with chlamydial urethritis will probably reduce the occurrence of this infection. Asymptomatic chlamydial infection in men and women responds to treatment, and the availability of new methods to identify these organisms will aid in this effort.

A single dose of tetracycline soon after sexual intercourse may be effective in preventing NGU, but this has not been studied conclusively.

In general, sexual intercourse should be avoided during symptomatic urethritis and also during treatment. Oral sex with a man with NGU might spread the organisms to the throat of the partner, but it is not clear if a symptomatic throat infection will develop. Any sexual partners of the past four weeks should be notified of their exposure so that they can seek appropriate treatment. Nonsexual close contact, such as intimate kissing and the sharing of food utensils, are not prohibited during an episode of nongonococcal urethritis.

4 / Vaginitis, Cervicitis, and Pelvic Inflammatory Disease

Vaginitis and Cervicitis

Vaginitis is one of the most common infections in sexually active women. Strictly speaking, not all episodes of vaginal infections are clearly sexually transmitted. Vaginitis itself means inflammation or irritation of the vagina, and may be due to a number of causes. But most cases of vaginitis are caused by one or more different organisms, and these infections can sometimes be transmitted sexually.

In general, three organisms or clusters of organisms are associated with vaginitis: *Trichomonas vaginalis; Candida albicans* or other yeastlike fungi; and the combination of the organism *Gardnerella vaginalis* and anaerobic bacteria (those which grow in the absence of oxygen).

The hallmark of vaginitis is the presence of an abnormal vaginal discharge. Normally, there is always some degree of vaginal fluid present, usually white or clear with flecks of material in the mucous substance. An abnormal discharge (known medically as leukorrhea) may be frothy and white, yellow, gray, brown, or greenish in color. There is often an unpleasant odor, and the quality of the material—usually dependent on the type of vaginitis—is most often homogeneous or smooth. These qualities alone, however, are rarely sufficient for a doctor to diagnose the causative organism. For example, the discharge associated with yeast infections, or candidiasis, is typically white, thick, and "cheesy" in character, but some women may have vaginitis due to these organisms without the characteristic discharge.

Cervicitis, or inflammation of the uterine cervix (the opening of the uterus that leads to the vagina), can be caused by herpes simplex virus, by *Chlamydia trachomatis*, or by *Neisseria gonorrhoeae*. These three organisms as well as *Trichomonas vaginalis* may also produce urethritis in men and in women (see Chapters 3 and 5), and herpes simplex virus can produce lesions occasionally in the vagina and frequently on the vulva (the external area of the female genitalia). The cells lining the cervix differ from those that line the vagina. Vaginal cells are not generally susceptible to infection with the gonococcal organism or with chlamydia, but cervical cells are.

Other symptoms associated with vaginitis include vaginal itching or vulvovaginal burning, pain and sometimes bleeding on intercourse, pain or burning on urination and increased urinary frequency, bleeding between periods, generalized discomfort or pelvic pain, rash, and occasional ulcers that often result from scratching.

Based on symptoms alone, differential diagnosis of cervicitis, vaginitis, and vulvovaginitis is difficult. Cervicitis may be present without any symptoms. Some women, however, may notice an unpleasant discharge as well as any of the above-mentioned symptoms of vaginitis. Symptoms similar to those described above can also be due to noninfectious causes. Irritation may be caused by a diaphragm, contraceptive foams, or such products as deodorants and douching materials. Occasionally vaginal irritation may result from masturbation, heavy sexual intercourse, or insertion of objects during sex play. Older women may develop vaginitis after menopause, most likely due to lower levels of estrogens and other female hormones. Some women may develop vaginitis or cervicitis as a result of using an intrauterine device (IUD). In these cases, the uterus itself may also be infected, and removal of the IUD, along with the use of intravenous antibiotics, is often necessary to eradicate this infection.

Diagnosis of cervicitis is usually made during a pelvic examination, when the physician can examine the cervix in detail. In addition, there are specific antibody stains and enzyme tests that allow rapid determination of the presence of chlamydia or herpes virus from a cervical swab. The gonococcal organism can be identified by a laboratory culture of the cervical mucus. Treatment of cervicitis is related to the infecting organism; see Gonorrhea, Chapter 1; Genital Herpes, Chapter 2; and Chlamydia, Chapter 3.

Trichomoniasis

Trichomonas vaginalis is a protozoal parasite. The details of how this organism causes vaginitis are not clear, but it probably excretes some toxin, or irritating product, which results in inflammation. The trichomonad organism can survive in the vagina for a long but undetermined amount of time and is readily transmissible by contact with the vagina or vaginal discharge. It can spread by way of the fingers or the penis, and possibly by such objects as douching equipment or vaginal applicators.

Men with trichomoniasis may reinfect their partner or transmit the organism to others during intercourse. Men exposed to the trichomonad may develop infections of the urethra, with or without symptoms, and possibly of the prostate gland (see Chapter 3).

Trichomonads cannot survive in the rectum and cause infection as a result of anal intercourse in women or men. A recent report suggests that trichomonads may be acquired from hot tubs.

Twenty to 30 percent of all women may have the trichomonad organism present, but not all will necessarily have symptoms. The typical trichomonad discharge is moderate in amount, may have an unpleasant odor, and may be gray, yellowish, or slightly bloody. Vaginal itching, pain on intercourse, and urinary-tract symptoms (increased urinary frequency, pain on voiding) may also occur. Sometimes there is chafing of the upper thighs caused by irritant material in the discharge.

Diagnosis of vaginitis due to *Trichomonas vaginalis* is usually made by examination of the vagina for a characteristic discharge and inflammation. Examination of a drop of vaginal fluid under the microscope will reveal the characteristically active moving organisms. This method is adequate in making a diagnosis in about 80 percent of the cases. A culture, however, is the best method for detecting the presence of the trichomonad, especially in nonsymptomatic patients. A doctor may also measure the acidity of the vaginal fluid, which is reduced in the presence of trichomonad infection. Pap smears may also be used in diagnosing trichomonad vaginitis.

Trichomonad vaginitis is best treated with metronidazole (Flagyl, Protostat, Satric), which is active against amoebas and bacteria normally present in the vagina. It is normally administered by mouth in a single dose of two grams. (Some studies suggest that one gram may be adequate.) Treatment with Flagyl vaginal suppositories for this infection is generally not adequate because the organism is often also present in the urethra and some of the glands around the urethra. Vaginal suppositories do not reach these areas, and symptoms will usually recur shortly after discontinuing the vaginal Flagyl suppository.

Flagyl has some minor side effects, including nausea, abdominal cramps, and diarrhea; a metallic taste may be present, and patients may experience nausea and vomiting after drinking alcoholic beverages while taking this drug.

Male sexual partners with or without obvious evidence of trichomoniasis should also be treated to prevent the Ping-Pong effect resulting in reinfection of female sexual partners. Usually single-dose treatment is also effective in men.

Metronidazole should not be used in the first trimester of pregnancy. Many physicians do not use it at all in pregnant women, to reduce the possible risk of fetal abnormalities or cancer; however, these risks have not been proved, but one study has suggested that Flagyl may impart an increased risk of stillborn and premature babies. *Trichomonas vaginalis* itself might colonize the vagina of female babies born of mothers with this infection, but this is usually not a serious problem. Women with vaginal infection due to trichomoniasis can achieve symptomatic relief with vinegar douches (two tablespoons of white vinegar in a quart of warm water). Some women are treated successfully during pregnancy with intravaginal clotrimazole (Lotrimin, Mycelex, and others). Sulfa-containing creams or suppositories are not effective in treating this infection. There are no known fetal effects of trichomonad infection. Breast milk of mothers who take metronidazole has been found to contain the drug, but the safety of this drug for use in nursing mothers has not been tested.

The use of oral contraceptives has not been associated with the risk of trichomonad infections. To the contrary, some studies suggest that oral contraceptives that provide extra estrogens may actually cause the vagina to be less susceptible to this infection.

Yeast Infection

Candida albicans is a yeastlike fungus responsible for a large number of episodes of vaginitis known as candidiasis, or monilia. Diagnosis of a vaginal yeast infection does not necessarily imply a sexually transmitted disease. On the other hand, the candida organism may produce a mild infection of the penis (especially around the indentation between the head and the shaft of the penis in uncircumcised men) in sexual partners of women with vaginal candida. Similarly, it has been suggested that vaginal candida infections are more frequent in women whose uncircumcised partners harbor this fungus under the foreskin.

Other species of candida and similar fungi may occasionally cause vaginitis. Yeastlike fungi can normally be cultured from the vagina in perhaps up to 30 percent of women. However, possibly a third of these have no vaginal symptoms. Yeastlike fungal infections are more frequent in women during pregnancy, in women taking oral contraceptive pills or antibiotics (especially broad-spectrum antibiotics), and in women with diabetes mellitus. The role of tight-fitting panty hose in the initiation of candidiasis is not clear. Many women, however, have noticed healing of this infection when panty hose are no longer used.

Vaginal itching is the major symptom associated with candidal infections of the vagina and may extend to the anal area. A white and curdlike vaginal discharge is usually present. Some women also complain of burning and stinging on urination, increased frequency of urination, and pain on intercourse. The vulva may appear reddened, and there may be a red, itchy rash in the area between the vulva and the thighs.

Diagnosis of candidal vaginitis may be made on microscopic examination of a drop of vaginal fluid, but the most effective means of proving this diagnosis is by culture of the discharge. Cultures usually yield a diagnosis within forty-eight hours but occasionally may take longer. Candidal infections increase the level of acidity of the vaginal fluid, a finding that is helpful in distinguishing yeastlike fungal infections from trichomonad vaginitis and nonspecific vaginitis.

Candidiasis can be successfully treated with a variety of medications. Many doctors use nystatin, clotrimazole, or miconazole vaginal suppositories. These drugs are also available in a cream that can be applied to the external genitalia and skin if inflammation is present. Male sexual partners with candidal yeast infection of the penis may respond well to nystatin or clotrimazole cream. Miconazole should not be used in the first trimester of pregnancy. Recently, gelatin capsules of boric-acid powder have been used successfully when inserted vaginally. This approach may be effective in preventing recurrences if used once or twice weekly.

Vaginal yeast infections do not usually affect pregnancy itself, although a few intrauterine infections have been reported. Babies born of mothers with yeast vaginitis may themselves be colonized and develop thrush or candidal diaper rash, but more serious infections are limited to premature babies.

There is a tendency for candidal vaginitis to recur. Sometimes recurrences are due to the presence of candida in the feces, and the simultaneous use of oral and intravaginal nystatin or other antifungal agents may be effective in preventing subsequent episodes of this type of infection. Oral nystatin is not well absorbed and therefore can be taken during pregnancy or during breast-feeding. Some physicians may use the new oral antifungal drug ketoconazole (Nizoral). This drug, although effective against vaginal candidiasis, should not be used during pregnancy or breast-feeding. Rarely, it may cause liver damage. Some physicians recommend reducing the fruit in one's diet; others recommend using a heat lamp to dry an infection that has spread to the thighs.

Nonspecific Vaginitis

"Nonspecific vaginitis" is a term applied to the appearance of an abnormal vaginal discharge that may have a fishy odor and may be associated with symptoms of vaginal itching, pain or burning on urination, and pain on intercourse in the absence of infection with *Trichomonas vaginalis* or *Candida albicans*. The cause of this condition has been the subject of much debate in the last ten or fifteen years. Originally it was ascribed to the organism known as *Corynebacterium vaginale*, also known as *Hemophilus vaginalis*. Most recently, this organism has been renamed *Gardnerella vaginalis*, after Dr. Herman Gardner, who popularized its association with vaginitis.

The problem is that *Gardnerella vaginalis* can be found normally in the vagina of women without any signs of vaginal irritation or infection. More recent investigations have suggested that this organism causes vaginitis only in the presence of other bacteria, of the Bacteroides species or similar anaerobic organisms. This condition also has been termed "bacterial vaginosis" because many women have this syndrome without real inflammation of the vaginal walls.

Gardnerella-associated or bacterial vaginosis is very common and may be present in about 30 percent of women attending clinics for sexually transmitted diseases. It may be more frequent in women who have had multiple pregnancies and in women with frequent sexual activity. Although it is not clearly sexually transmitted, it is highly likely that about 70 percent of male sexual partners of women with this infection will have *Gardnerella vaginalis* cultivated from their urethra. Oral-contraceptive use may also be associated with increased risk of this infection.

Nonspecific vaginitis, or bacterial vaginosis, is suspected by a physician if a gray discharge is present. Diagnosis is based on an examination of this material, revealing the presence of so-called clue cells. These cells are identified under the microscope as being packed with small bacteria believed to be *Gardnerella vaginalis*. Microscopic examination may also reveal a decrease in the number of normal vaginal bacteria (lactobacilli) and a relative increase in the organisms believed to be *Gardnerella vaginalis*.

Mixing a small amount of vaginal fluid with potassium hydroxide solution can help confirm the diagnosis if a fishy odor results. This odor is due to the presence of volatile amines, malodorous chemicals released during multiplication of certain anaerobic bacteria. Some chemical analyses of vaginal fluids have also demonstrated the presence of these amines confirming the diagnosis. This technique, however, is not generally available in most laboratories.

Women who have nonspecific vaginitis or bacterial vaginosis may be somewhat predisposed to developing cervicitis (usually due to *Chlamydia trachomatis*), or they may develop uterine infection due to mycoplasma or other organisms.

Treatment of nonspecific vaginitis in nonpregnant women is generally with metronidazole (Flagyl). In this type of vaginitis, however, the drug must be taken several times a day for a week to work against the anaerobic bacteria and ultimately cure the infection; it is not active against the *Gardnerella* organism. Flagyl should be avoided during pregnancy and while breast-feeding. Ampicillin and a few other antibiotics have had some success in treating pregnant women, however. There are no known fetal effects of nonspecific vaginitis in pregnancy.

Sulfonamide creams or suppositories are much less effective, if at all. It is not clear yet whether nonsymptomatic male sexual partners need to be treated to reduce reinfection of the female partner.

General Prevention of Vaginitis and Cervicitis

Condom use can reduce transmission of gonorrhea and those infections due to chlamydia and trichomoniasis. Treatment of all sexual partners for trichomonad infection can also help prevent a recurrence. Frequency of vaginitis, as with all sexually transmitted diseases, is lessened when the number of sexual partners is reduced.

With respect to trichomonad infections, sharing towels, douching equipment, and sexual objects can serve as means of transmission of this parasite. Nonoxynol-9 contraceptive jellies and foams are, in fact, lethal to the trichomonad organism when tested in vitro, but the routine use of these products for this purpose is not recommended because of the lack of clinical success.

Sexual transmission of the yeastlike fungus infections is not as clearly defined as for other organisms. For women with frequent and severe vaginal fungus infections, recurrences can perhaps be minimized by avoiding tight-fitting panty hose and possibly by using prophylactic vaginal antifungal agents during broad-spectrum-antibiotic treatments for other infections.

Many women are found to have more than one of these infecting organisms simultaneously. Thus, in order to completely eradicate the symptoms of vaginitis and cervicitis, treatment must often be aimed at more than one causative organism.

Pelvic Inflammatory Disease

Pelvic inflammatory disease (PID), known medically as salpingitis, is a common term for inflammation of the fallopian tubes in the female reproductive system. It usually represents the ascent of infection from the cervix through the uterus and into the fallopian tubes.

Many different organisms can cause pelvic inflammatory disease. The importance of each organism varies considerably from country to country. In the United States the organism of gonorrhea, aerobic and anaerobic bacteria, *Chlamydia trachomatis,* and *Mycoplasma hominis* are important causes. Mycoplasmas are bacteria that lack cell walls and can cause infection in the lung, the middle ear, and the genital tract. There are two major types of genital mycoplasmas: *Mycoplasma hominis* and *Ureaplasma urealyticum.* Some women have infections caused by more than one of these organisms.

PID is quite common and occurs in varying degrees of severity in about one million women per year in the United States. It is one of the more serious complications of many sexually transmitted diseases, including gonorrhea, cervicitis, and urethritis.

The complications of pelvic inflammatory disease can

include sterility due to scarring of the fallopian tubes. Ectopic pregnancies, or fertilized eggs implanted in one of the fallopian tubes rather than in the uterus, may also result from this scarring. Some women, if not treated promptly, may develop pelvic abscesses affecting the tube and the ovary. Some women may develop chronic-pelvic-pain syndrome, presumably associated with residual adhesions as a result of the inflammatory process in the tubes.

It is not known why some women develop PID and why others do not given the same sexually transmitted disease. It seems clear, however, that having multiple sexual partners and using an IUD enhance the risk of pelvic inflammatory disease. PID is more frequent in women under thirty who use an IUD. The incidence of PID may be somewhat lower in women who use oral-contraceptive pills, possibly because of decreased contractile activity of the uterus associated with these drugs.

Pelvic inflammatory disease usually causes fever, lower pelvic or abdominal pain, and often a vaginal discharge. A doctor can confirm this diagnosis if there is pain when the cervix is manipulated and if pain and tenderness are felt in the area of the ovaries and the fallopian tubes. Some physicians may examine the tubes and the ovaries directly by means of a laparoscope. This is a small fiberoptic tube that is inserted through the lower abdominal wall and allows for a complete visual examination of the infected structures and collection of specimens for culture. In addition, some physicians may perform a needle aspiration through the vagina into the area behind the uterus to collect pus from the infected tubes, thereby allowing for a definitive diagnosis by culture and optimal selection of antibiotic therapy.

Other conditions that may mimic pelvic inflammatory disease include ectopic pregnancy, appendicitis, pending rupture of an ovarian cyst, and endometriosis.

Fortunately, most women with PID respond to effective therapy, which can be achieved with a variety of antibiotics administered intravenously in severe cases and orally in milder ones. Early treatment is likely to prevent major complications, but PID can recur, especially in women who have strictures or other abnormalities of the fallopian tubes caused by the initial infection. Once the cause of an episode of PID has been determined, all sexual partners should be treated appropriately. This will help minimize reinfection and recurrence of this disease.

5 / Urinary-Tract Infections in Women

Urinary-tract infections are not sexually transmitted diseases. However, symptoms of this type of infection often occur in the genital area, and many women associate recurrences of this infection with sexual activity. Urinary-tract infections are among the most common infections known, second only to the common cold. About 25 percent of all women have at least one episode of urinary-tract infection during their lifetime, and at any one point about 5 percent of all women will have some evidence of an active infection.

Urinary infections are common in women during pregnancy and may increase in frequency with advancing age. Infections of the urinary tract are considerably less common in men, possibly because the shorter and straighter female urethra (the tube that transports urine from the bladder) is more likely to allow entrance of infecting organisms.

Asymptomatic and acute symptomatic urinary infections during pregnancy have been associated with the increased risk of low-birth-weight and premature babies, fetal distress, and deformities in the newborn. Routine medical screening for nonsymptomatic bacterial infections during pregnancy can reduce such risks.

It is often very difficult to determine whether the infection is limited to the lower urinary tract (urethra and bladder) or to the upper urinary tract (kidney and collecting system). Symptoms of urethritis (inflammation of the urethra) are virtually identical to those of cystitis (inflammation of the urinary bladder). Some women with vaginitis (see Chapter 4) may have similar symptoms without actual infection in the urinary tract. While some women have only a single bout of acute urethritis, cystitis, or pyelonephritis (infection of the kidney and its collecting ducts), others may have as many as ten or twenty such infections per year. Some women develop chronic or continual infections of the urinary tract, but these women form a very small minority and often have kidney stones or some other structural abnormality of the urinary tract.

It is not clearly known why some women are subject to frequent or recurrent urinary-tract infections while others are not. Recent evidence suggests that the cells lining the urethra, and possibly the area around the urethra and in the vagina, are slightly different in those women who are subject to these infections. There may be a correlation between these cellular differences and the ability of the infecting organisms to adhere to these cells as a first step in the infectious process. Research in this area may lead to a means of blocking this adherence mechanism in some way.

Many different types of infecting organisms may cause the symptoms associated with urinary-tract infections. Most patients with cystitis and infection of the kidney are infected with common bacteria, usually *Escherichia coli*, Proteus species, or other similar bacteria. These organisms are normally present in the feces and are frequently found around the anus. Women who are subject to recurrent urinary-tract infections due to bacteria often have these organisms present in the vagina or in the area around the urethral opening prior to infection.

Bacteria produce symptoms by virtue of their ability to irritate and inflame the lining of the bladder or the urethra. When bacteria multiply, as they do in the urine during infection, they produce a variety of products that irritate these structures.

Other organisms may produce infection that is limited to the urethra. These include *Chlamydia trachomatis*, *Trichomonas vaginalis*, and *Neisseria gonorrhoeae*, the organism that causes gonorrhea. The virus that causes genital herpes may also produce symptoms of urethritis due to irritation of a blister or vesicle in the area of the urethra. Other bacteria such as *Staphylococcus saprophyticus* may also cause urethritis.

It is unlikely that sexual activity per se causes urinary-tract infections. These infections certainly occur in sexually inactive women. It has been demonstrated that bacteria can be introduced into the urethra and the bladder during sexual intercourse, but these bacteria are present in very small numbers. The normal voiding and defense mechanisms of the bladder appear to eliminate these organisms before they establish an infection.

Some women, however, clearly relate recurrence or exacerbation of urinary-tract infections with sexual intercourse, particularly heavy sexual activity. Although the penis does not usually penetrate the urethra during sexual activity, the thrusting activity just below can cause some irritation and trauma to the urinary opening and result in the introduction of bacteria into the bladder. Sexual activity may also exacerbate the problem in women who already have the causative organisms present in the urethra and who are prone to developing urinary infection. This form of sexually related infection can be prevented (see below).

It is not clear why *Chlamydia trachomatis* causes urethritis in some women, but the organism is known to be present in the cervix of 5 to 20 percent of sexually active women and is also known to cause urethritis in men. It is sexually transmitted from the cervix, possibly by entering the urethra by way of the vagina.

SYMPTOMS

Urinary-tract infection can be present without any symptoms. Known as asymptomatic bacteriuria, it may be associated with the eventual development of symptoms, or it may disappear spontaneously. The occurrence of asymptomatic bacteriuria in women increases with age and probably affects about 1 percent of all female children and teenagers. This figure rises about 1 percent for every ten years of age during the childbearing years, and as many as 15 percent of women over sixty-five may have asymptomatic bacteriuria.

When the urinary tract is infected, any part may be involved. For example, the infection may be limited to the urethra, the bladder itself, or the kidney and its collecting ducts. Regardless of the location and level of infection, most patients have similar symptoms, at least at the onset of infection. Bladder infection may spread to the kidneys, and renal infection may spread to the bloodstream. Occasionally, a long-term untreated kidney infection may result in permanent damage to the kidneys.

Common symptoms include burning or stinging on urination, increased frequency or urgency of urination, frequent waking during the night to urinate, and involuntary urination (stress incontinence). In addition, some women experience pain in the pelvic area over the bladder, and in some cases blood may be present in the urine. This does not necessarily indicate a more serious infection. Women who have infections in the kidney and its collecting system are more likely to experience fever, chills, back or side pain, nausea, and vomiting, although these symptoms are not always present when the kidney is involved.

DIAGNOSIS

A physician can make a definitive diagnosis of urinary-tract infection from the results of a urine culture. Bacteria that cause cystitis and pyelonephritis can be cultivated from the urine in a bacteriology laboratory. The culture specimen must be a "clean-voided" one. You should first cleanse the area around the opening of the urethra with three or four washes of soap solution. Then spread the lips of the vagina and void directly into a clean, dry collecting cup without touching the cup to your body. This urine should then be covered and refrigerated or sent to the laboratory for immediate processing.

Part of the urine sample will be cultured for specific

bacteria, which will take one or two days, and the remainder will be evaluated by urinalysis. Urinalysis simply tests for inflammatory cells, blood cells, and other constituents such as sugar and protein. White blood cells found in the urine suggest infection but do not identify the type of infecting organism or the location.

Women with frequent or recurrent urinary infections are often infected with different strains of bacteria with each occurrence. Those who are recurrently infected with the same bacterial strain are more likely to have infection in the upper urinary tract or kidney. In these cases a detailed study of the urinary tract with X rays of the kidney may be necessary to determine the best treatment.

Some women develop recurrent urinary-tract infections (especially those infections that are difficult to control with antibiotics) due to some mild abnormality in the urethral structure, impairing the flow of urine from the bladder to the urethral opening. These women may benefit from urological evaluation which might include an intravenous pyelogram, an X-ray study of the urinary tract after voiding, or a study of the flow patterns of urination.

The diagnosis of chlamydial urethritis is usually made by ruling out other known bacterial causes through laboratory culture. Chlamydial cultures are not routinely available in most laboratories, but new and simple techniques for the detection of these organisms have been introduced recently.

On occasion a physician may need to perform a bladder tap, or aspiration, if the bacterial cultures on voided urine are difficult to evaluate. This process involves the placement of a thin needle directly into the bladder through the abdominal wall after anesthetizing the skin. Samples of the bladder urine obtained in this way help distinguish between urethral contamination and bladder infection.

TREATMENT

Most urinary-tract infections respond well to treatment. The bacteria responsible for causing first episodes of urinary-tract infection are usually susceptible to a wide variety of commonly used antibiotics. Most of these antibiotics can be administered by mouth and appear in the urine in very high concentrations. Frequently used antimicrobial agents for this infection include such sulfa drugs as Gantrisin or Gantanol, or ampicillin, amoxicillin, cephalexin, tetracycline, nitrofurantoin (Macrodantin) among others. Trimethroprim-sulfamethoxazole (Bactrim or Septra) is also used by many physicians.

Antibiotics used to be administered for seven to ten days, but recent studies suggest that a single high dose of an antibiotic by mouth may be effective in eradicating uncomplicated bacterial infections in the urine. Single-dose therapy is not effective in treating infections of the kidney or recurrent infections with the same organism, which usually require long-term treatment. Women with acute pyelonephritis are often quite ill and may need to be hospitalized and treated with intravenous antibiotics.

Women with frequent recurrent urinary-tract infections may benefit from so-called long-term suppressive treatment, which involves taking small doses of an antimicrobial agent every night or every other night to decrease the likelihood of bacteria multiplying and causing infection. This type of treatment is effective but must be continued over several years. Long-term side effects are usually uncommon, but your doctor should monitor for these with occasional examinations and blood tests.

Women with frequent infections that seem to be associated with sexual intercourse or menstruation may also benefit from the prophylactic use of a low dose of an antibiotic at these times. A single dose of an appropriate antibiotic just after intercourse will almost always prevent symptomatic infection. Frequent urine cultures over several years should be obtained to be certain that bladder urine has not become infected with a resistant strain of bacteria.

Most physicians recommend drinking large amounts of fluid during the treatment of urinary infections. This is thought to dilute the toxic or irritating products of bacterial multiplication. Once the antibiotics have had their effect on the bacteria in a day or so, "pushing fluids" is not really necessary. Other special diets are not necessary, although vitamin C (ascorbic acid) in large doses (about four grams a day) may have some antibacterial effect in the urine.

One can still engage in sexual activities while being treated for a urinary infection. If symptoms are present, however, it might be more comfortable to refrain from sex until treatment has had an effect.

PREVENTION

Since the actual cause of urinary-tract infections in women who are prone to them has not been determined, it is difficult to recommend effective ways of prevention. Good hygiene, while recommended, is not guaranteed to prevent these infections.

There is no evidence that diaphragm use, frequent douching, or bubble baths cause urinary-tract infection. Some women, however, may experience irritation of the urethral opening as a result of these products. If so, the use of the products should be discontinued. Many physicians suggest that women who have recurrent urinary-tract infections especially after intercourse should empty their bladder immediately following sex. The efficacy of this procedure has not been proved, but it is unlikely to cause harm. Most symptomatic episodes of infection in women who are prone to recurrences can be prevented by the long-term suppressive therapy outlined above.

Cranberry juice has been touted for years as a possible preventive for urinary-tract infections. Cranberries do contain an organic acid that can inhibit bacterial multiplication, but the substance is present in such small amounts in ordinary cranberry-juice cocktail that one may need to drink gallons of it for any documented biological effect to occur. However, there is no harm in drinking cranberry juice, and whole cranberry sauce does contain a fair amount of this acid; even so, it might require two or three cans a day to successfully treat or prevent urinary-tract infections.

6 / Syphilis

Although the disease was named syphilis only in the sixteenth century, it was probably known to the ancient
Chinese two or three thousand years before Christ. There
are numerous Biblical references to diseases that most likely
were forms of syphilis. It is alleged, for instance, that an
ancient Egyptian pharaoh acquired syphilis from Abraham's
wife, Sarah. In Genesis (12:17) we read, "And the Lord
plagued Pharaoh and his house with great plagues because
of Sarah, Abraham's wife." David also may have suffered
from syphilis, and it is alleged that he contracted it from
Bathsheba in that their child was "very sick": "And it came
to pass on the seventh day, that the child died" (2 Samuel
12:18). Some of David's lamentations also imply that he
had syphilis. From Psalms (38:3) we read: "There is no
soundness in my flesh because of my sin. . . . My wounds
stink, and are corrupt. . . . For my loins are filled with
loathsome disease. . . . My lovers and my friends stand
aloof from my sore; and my kinsmen stand afar off."

Much of what is assumed to be leprosy in the Bible and in medieval times was actually syphilis. There are probable references to syphilis in the writings of Hippocrates, Galen, Celsus, and Pliny.

Syphilis in the Bible and early times was associated with orgiastic behavior and debauchery in the grand style. Greeks and Romans worshiped the god Priapus (the medical term "priapism" survives today and refers to persistent erection of the penis), and a cult of ancient Hebrews who worshiped a similar god, Baal-Peor, was associated with prostitution and presumed syphilis. Moses, who had outlawed prostitution, warred with the Midianites, who worshiped Baal-Peor. The Plague of Baal-Peor is said to have been syphilis, and Moses, being a radical practitioner of public health, ordered the slaying of all women known to have practiced prostitution.

Syphilis received its name in a poem by the Italian poet Girolamo Fracastoro in 1530, and it derives from the Greek meaning companion of love. Fracastoro's poem was entitled "Syphilis sive Morbus Gallicus," meaning "Syphilis or the French Disease." In the sixteenth century, the Italians referred to syphilis as the French disease; the French called it the Italian disease; the Germans called it the French pox; the Dutch called it the Spanish disease; the Japanese called it the Portuguese disease, and so on, reflecting the turbulent history of invasions in this period.

Syphilis is caused by the bacterium spirochete *Treponema pallidum*, which is a coiled or spirallike organism. However, it was once thought to be caused by the same agent that caused gonorrhea. In 1767, in an attempt to prove that this was not the case, John Hunter, an English physician and anatomist, inoculated himself with pus from a patient who had a classical case of gonorrhea. Unfortunately, Hunter developed both diseases, as the patient who provided the pus also had undiagnosed syphilis.

Today syphilis remains a common disease. With the introduction of penicillin, however, there has been a dramatic decrease in the incidence of this disease, especially since World War II. In 1955, reported syphilis in the United States was at an all-time low of four out of every one hundred thousand people. However, with changes in sexual practices and the introduction of oral contraception, syphilis, like gonorrhea, was born again. There are about thirty thousand cases of syphilis reported annually in the United States today, making this the third most frequently *reported* infectious disease, following chicken pox and gonorrhea. (Other STDs, including nongonococcal urethritis and genital herpes, are considerably more frequent, but the law does not require that these be reported.) In the past five years there has been only a slight, but steady, rise in the number of reported cases of primary and secondary syphilis.

Most cases of syphilis develop in large metropolitan areas. More than 60 percent of the cases reported in 1981 were from sixty-three cities with populations of more than two hundred thousand, which represents only 26 percent of the American population. The number of cases reported in women attending both private and public STD services has remained reasonably constant in recent years. The occurrence of syphilis in white men attending public and private STD services, however, has increased gradually over the past fifteen years and more sharply over the past five years. Homosexually active men account for a disproportionately large number of the increased cases in recent years, and may account for about half of the cases in the United States today. This is most likely due to the fact that syphilis in the anal-rectal area may produce no obvious symptoms and may therefore be unknowingly transmitted to an active partner during anal intercourse. In fact, many people know they have some disease only when the symptoms of secondary syphilis develop.

Syphilis, today, is usually seen and treated in its early stages as a genital sore before progressing any further. It has been known as "the great masquerader," because it can, in its later stages, produce a wide variety of symptoms, some of which can mimic other diseases. The distinguished turn-of-the-century physician William Osler is said to have stated, "He who knows syphilis knows medicine." Untreated, syphilis develops in three stages: early, latent, and late syphilis. *Early syphilis* includes primary and secondary syphilis. It first manifests as a primary lesion, or chancre, and then produces symptoms of secondary syphilis. Following the symptoms of secondary syphilis, there is a *latent period* of up to twenty to thirty years after the initial infection. If there are any recurrences of the disease, they generally occur within the first two to four years after the initial infection. Following the latent phase; *tertiary* or *late syphilis* may develop in about 30 to 40 percent of untreated patients. The use of penicillin and other antibiotics has greatly decreased the number of people who develop late syphilis.

Syphilis is transmitted by close intimate or sexual contact with infectious lesions. Since most of the primary lesions of syphilis occur on the genitals, the vast majority (well over

95 percent) of cases are acquired by sexual contact. Syphilis can also be transmitted via lesions on the lips or in the throat. The *Treponema pallidum* organism usually infects mucous membranes more readily than intact skin. However, it is likely that the organism can enter through skin abrasions or possibly at the base of hair follicles on unbroken skin. After it enters the skin, it multiplies and produces the local primary lesion. The organisms may then enter the bloodstream via the lymphatic system.

Syphilis is rarely transmitted by blood transfusions; donated blood is routinely screened for evidence of syphilis, and any undetected *Treponema pallidum* organisms in donated blood usually die within three or four days of blood-bank refrigeration. A contaminated needle can transmit the infection, but this is quite rare. The skin and mucous-membrane lesions of congenital syphilis are highly contagious; infection can be spread by close contact with any of these lesions.

Some degree of immunity to reinfection does exist in people with syphilis; it is unlikely for a person to become infected a second time during the primary or subsequent phases of untreated syphilis. However, once early syphilis has been treated, the treated individual is again susceptible to reinfections if reexposed to a partner with active syphilis.

Homosexually active men with multiple sexual partners are at special risk of acquiring syphilis. The frequency of nonsymptomatic syphilitic lesions occurring in the anus and the rectum is not clearly known, but blood-test screening in gay bathhouses in Denver and Los Angeles discovered that 1 to 3 percent of patrons had previously undetected infection with syphilis. A marked reduction in the number of new cases of syphilis in gay men has been reported recently in New York, probably reflecting a change in sexual practices as a reaction to the increasing occurrence of the acquired immunodeficiency syndrome (AIDS).

Not everyone who comes in contact with an infectious lesion of syphilis will develop the disease. The risk of disease increases with the number of organisms present in the lesion. Primary chancres and the lesions of secondary syphilis are highly infectious, however.

Congenital Syphilis

Syphilis can be transmitted at any time during pregnancy from the mother to the fetus. However, the risk of transmission becomes greater the later (particularly after four months) syphilis is acquired during pregnancy.

Most obstetrical facilities routinely screen for the presence of syphilis by means of a blood test early in pregnancy. However, very few such services routinely reexamine women later in pregnancy and at the time of delivery. As a result, pregnant women who are incubating syphilis (when the blood tests may still prove negative) and those who acquire syphilis later in pregnancy (after the initial blood test) are still at risk of transmitting this infection to the fetus. Women who think they may have been exposed to syphilis during pregnancy should consult their physicians and request blood tests for themselves and their newborn.

There are many possible manifestations of congenital

syphilis, and they may appear in infancy or during childhood. Some infants may be totally unaffected. Others are born with an enlarged liver and enlarged lymph nodes, pneumonia, anemia and other blood problems, skin rash, jaundice, abnormalities and inflammation of the bones, kidney disease, central-nervous-system disorders, inflammation of the eyes, or inflammation of the pancreas. Infants may be born prematurely or have a low birth weight. In addition, the placenta may show abnormal aspects consistent with congenital syphilis. Some of the skin lesions, if present, may contain the *Treponema pallidum* organisms. Severely ill infants are sometimes misdiagnosed because other infections can produce similar problems in the newborn.

Some of the manifestations of congenital syphilis may not develop until later in the first two years of life. In addition, not all of the above manifestations may be present in any one infant at any one time. Unfortunately, because classical symptoms, including runny nose, blisterlike rashes on the palms or soles, and enlargement of the spleen, do not always appear, physicians may overlook syphilis as the cause of problems in newborns.

Later in childhood as bones, joints, and skin mature, other problems may occur for the first time. For example, deformities in the skeletal system, including the palate, nasal bones, tibia (shin bone), collarbone, shoulder bone, or teeth, may occur. Older children with congenital syphilis may become deaf or slightly retarded, develop such eye problems as scarring of the corneas, or have seizures and paralysis of various muscles. Linear scarring of the upper lip (rhagades) may also occur. Certain forms of congenital heart disease have been linked to congenital syphilis.

SYMPTOMS

The primary lesion of syphilis is the chancre. It begins as a small pimple, or papule, that gradually enlarges, erodes, and ultimately forms an ulcer. The ulcer is usually painless, and its edges tend to be somewhat firm and raised. It has the appearance of a "punched-out" area, with the base of the ulcer being somewhat red. On occasion more than one chancre may appear, and they may also appear atypical and cause pain, mimicking herpes or chancroid. The lymph nodes that drain the involved area may become enlarged and feel slightly tender. The primary chancre can occur at almost any body site if contact occurs between a heavily infected lesion and a somewhat abraded area of skin, but the genital areas are the most common. These syphilitic ulcers typically appear on the shaft or the base of the penis, or in the vagina, the anus, the rectum, or the mouth.

The primary lesion develops anywhere from one week to three months after direct contact with an infectious syphilitic lesion of another person, with the average lesion developing three weeks after contact. Only about 50 percent of the sexual partners of a person with syphilis will develop the infection. Lesions situated deep in the vagina or the throat or in the rectum may not produce any other symptoms and, therefore, may not be noticed. In these instances syphilis can easily be spread to sexual partners unknowingly. This is one reason why highly sexually active people should have routine examinations of all sexually involved sites at least once every six months. People who have had previous attacks of syphilis should be carefully examined, because recurrences may produce an atypical primary lesion that may in fact be syphilis.

The chancre normally disappears and heals spontaneously by six weeks after its initial appearance. A slight scar may remain at this site. Treatment can usually accelerate this healing process. When syphilis occurs in the mouth, the throat, the rectum, or the anus, it may be joined by infection from other bacteria normally present at these sites.

If the primary lesion is not treated, manifestations of secondary syphilis may develop. This stage of the disease is extremely varied in its symptoms and may mimic a wide variety of other diseases.

Secondary syphilis usually develops six to eight weeks after the primary lesion disappears, but some of the secondary manifestations may occur while the primary lesion is still present. Most people develop a generalized or widespread skin rash that usually consists of flat, red or pink spots or bumps, which may develop on the arms, the chest, or the back and then spread to most areas of the body. The rash typically involves the palms of the hands and the soles of the feet, a feature that often helps physicians recognize this disease. Some patches of discolored mucous membrane may occur in such moist areas as the lips, the mouth, or the vagina.

Some form of generalized illness, such as fever, malaise, some loss of appetite, or swelling of the lymph glands, may occur at the onset of secondary syphilis. These symptoms resemble those of infectious mononucleosis, among other diseases. Weight loss, joint pains, sore throat, or laryngitis may also occur, but these symptoms by themselves rarely indicate the presence of syphilis.

People with secondary syphilis may also lose their hair in areas of the scalp or the beard or the outer part of the eyebrows or eyelashes. Many other symptoms may develop, with such rare serious complications as meningitis, hepatitis, or kidney or bone disease. Symptoms of the nervous system are uncommon even though neurological involvement with syphilis may be present in about one-third of those with secondary syphilis. Almost any organ of the body can be affected during this stage. All of the lesions of secondary syphilis are extremely infectious and contagious.

Today, most people with primary and secondary syphilis are treated effectively (see below), and as a result later forms of syphilis have become extremely rare. However, if the disease is left untreated, latent syphilis develops, which is divided into the early and late phases. The early latent phase may last up to four years after infection, with no specific symptoms. However, the blood test remains positive and people continue to be somewhat infectious.

The late latent phase may never produce any symptoms. In general, late latent syphilis is not infectious except in the case of pregnant women who may transmit syphilis to their fetus during pregnancy.

Late syphilis, the last stage of untreated syphilis, may produce lesions in the heart and the blood vessels, in the brain and the nervous system, or occasionally in the liver, the bones, or other organs.

Lesions affecting the heart and the blood vessels occur in about one out of ten untreated patients with syphilis, and often develop fifteen to twenty years after the initial syphilitic lesion. Therefore, most people with late syphilis do not even remember having ever had a genital or other primary lesion. This form of syphilis involves weakening of certain blood vessels in and around the heart and may lead to death. Fortunately, this form of syphilis is seen very rarely today.

Manifestations of late syphilis affecting the nervous system occur even later than those affecting the heart and the blood vessels and may occur up to twenty-five or more years after the initial infection. Many of those with late syphilis of the nervous system do not develop any symptoms, and for this reason most physicians will perform spinal taps on those who have an unexplained positive blood test for syphilis. Spinal taps can determine the presence or absence of nonsymptomatic neurosyphilis, and effective treatment for this condition can prevent the development of symptoms. On the other hand, people who do have symptoms of central-nervous-system syphilis may develop a variety of problems including seizures or convulsions, weakness and difficulty in walking, impotence, difficulty in urinating, shooting pains in the back and the legs, a variety of problems with weight-bearing joints, visual defects, vertigo, and, rarely, deafness.

All of the manifestations of secondary, latent, and late syphilis can be completely prevented by effectively treating the initial chancre.

DIAGNOSIS

Diagnosis of syphilis is usually made by examination of the lesions and either microscopic examination of the typical spirochetes in a sample taken from the skin lesion (during the primary phase) or by a blood test (during secondary syphilis).

Blood tests for syphilis have undergone considerable refinement in recent years, and more accurate methods are likely to become available. However, at present the blood test is not a very sensitive test for detecting the primary or early stage of syphilis. Two major types of blood tests are available: the nonspecific tests and those which detect the presence of antibodies to the *Treponema pallidum* organism itself. The nonspecific, or nontreponemal, serological blood test for syphilis (also known as the Wassermann or VDRL test) is performed most frequently. This test is positive in only about 60 percent of people with early or primary syphilis, but will become positive in almost all cases by four or five weeks after the chancre develops. This test, as well as other blood tests, is positive in virtually all people with secondary syphilis.

The nontreponemal blood test is also very useful in following the effects of treatment. It will generally become negative by one year after effective treatment of primary or secondary syphilis. In patients with untreated syphilis, this test may become negative after many years, even in the absence of treatment.

On the other hand, the specific treponemal test may remain positive for life, since it measures the presence of antibodies to syphilis in the bloodstream. This type of test may be used to verify the result of a false positive nontreponemal test.

Positive nontreponemal tests may falsely indicate syphilis in women during pregnancy, in drug addicts, in the elderly, and in people who have such diseases as lupus and rheumatoid arthritis. False positive tests for syphilis may also occur if a person has another infectious disease such as malaria, chicken pox, measles, other spirochetal infections, leprosy, tuberculosis, hepatitis, mononucleosis, and occasionally the common cold. False positive tests can be further evaluated with a specific treponemal antibody test.

The *Treponema pallidum* organism cannot be cultivated routinely on artificial media. Thus one cannot request a culture for syphilis. The organism can be cultivated in animals, however. Although rabbits have been used for this purpose in the past, most modern laboratories no longer use live animals to test for the presence of this organism. The *Treponema pallidum* organism is quite fragile and dies in twenty-four to forty-eight hours when exposed to oxygen, high or low temperatures, or drying.

TREATMENT

All phases and stages of syphilis are treatable. The drug of choice is penicillin, but tetracycline and erythromycin are also effective. Although the *Treponema pallidum* spirochete is very sensitive to penicillin, adequate levels of this drug must be taken over a ten-day to two-week period.

People who have had syphilis for more than one year without treatment probably should have a spinal tap to rule out the presence of nonsymptomatic neurosyphilis, which requires longer treatment with higher doses to successfully eradicate the disease. Pregnant women with syphilis can be treated with penicillin or erythromycin, and babies with congenital syphilis should be treated with penicillin in doses appropriate to the stage or type of syphilis present.

Blood tests should be repeated three, six, and twelve months after treatment, to follow the effect of the treatment program. People who have had syphilis for more than one year should have an additional blood test two years after treatment. Retreatment may be necessary in some cases.

Those who have been exposed to infectious primary syphilis as a result of sexual contact (even if it has already been three months) should also receive diagnostic evaluation and treatment for presumed syphilis, even if there are no symptoms yet present. With secondary syphilis, all sexual contacts within the past year should be referred for treatment.

PREVENTION

Syphilis may be prevented by using a condom, but this method of prophylaxis only prevents transmission from, or to, those genital sites that are actually covered by the condom. A primary chancre may occur at the base of the shaft of the penis in an area not covered by the condom. Similarly, a lesion on the lip or the tongue may result from direct contact with an infected area during oral sex. Using a condom will definitely decrease the risk of acquiring syphilis, but using a diaphragm will not offer the same protection to women.

People who think they might have the primary or secondary form of this disease should refrain from sexual activity or any close intimate contact until they are diagnosed and receive treatment.

Contact-tracing and treatment of people known to have had sexual contact with any person with diagnosed syphilis can dramatically reduce the spread of this disease. This procedure involves confidential personal interviews with the diagnosed patient and all of his or her recent sexual contacts. It is quite important, therefore, for people who acquire syphilis to inform their previous sexual partners of their exposure and to advise them to seek prompt therapy even in the absence of any symptoms. The routine use of antibiotics after sexual exposure as a preventive measure is not recommended unless it is known that the partner is, or has been, infected with syphilis, in which case full treatment is necessary.

Screening of pregnant women early and late in pregnancy or at the time of delivery by means of a blood test for syphilis has reduced the number of cases of congenital syphilis. In addition, the routine screening of blood in the umbilical cord would allow the detection of syphilis in newborns. Syphilis is not usually transmitted in breast milk, but if a primary chancre or secondary skin lesion is present on the nipple or the breast, syphilis could be transmitted to the nursing infant.

By law, all cases of syphilis must be reported to the health department. This is usually done by a doctor at the time of diagnosis. All information is used in the strictest confidence to facilitate contact-tracing and to control the spread of this infection. These records are not made available to any public or private source.

7 / Hepatitis

Hepatitis is inflammation of the liver. The term "hepatitis" does not necessarily imply sexually transmitted disease or, for that matter, any infection. Hepatitis can result from an infectious as well as a noninfectious cause. Some of the noninfectious causes include alcohol, hormones, and toxins.

Of the viruses associated with hepatitis, the three most common are hepatitis A, hepatitis B, and non-A non-B. The viruses may cause similar symptoms, but they are often acquired in different ways.

Hepatitis can also be caused by cytomegalovirus (CMV), the virus of infectious mononucleosis (also known as the Epstein-Barr virus), the herpes simplex virus, and the virus of German measles. Hepatitis may also result from the bacteria that causes gonorrhea and by the agent of nongonococcal urethritis, *Chlamydia trachomatis*. (In these latter two cases hepatitis often manifests as an inflammation around the liver associated with pelvic inflammatory disease in women, although it has also been described in men.) Syphilis rarely causes hepatitis.

Hepatitis A

Hepatitis-A infection is also known as infectious hepatitis or short-incubation hepatitis. Traditionally it has been spread by means of contaminated shellfish, food, or drinking water. Hepatitis A is often seen in institutions for the mentally ill, or in schools for retarded children, or in day-care facilities in which contact with feces contaminated with hepatitis-A virus can occur. Hepatitis A is also known to spread in families of patients who have the disease. Since the hepatitis-A virus is shed into the stool for up to three weeks before the illness produces symptoms, it can also be transmitted sexually by oral–anal intercourse. This route of infection with hepatitis-A virus is quite common, even following careful cleansing or rectal douching. Hepatitis A is not thought to be transmitted by vaginal intercourse or genital–anal intercourse. This virus is rarely transmitted by contact with blood or transfusion of blood products.

Hepatitis A is quite common in the general population. Antibodies to this virus, indicating previous exposure, are found in approximately 40 percent of American adults. Antibodies may be present even in those who have never had any symptoms of the disease. The infection occurs at a much higher rate in those of lower socioeconomic status, with rates as high as 60 percent occurring among the poor.

Hepatitis-A virus has been isolated only recently and is clearly different from hepatitis-B virus. Hepatitis-A virus is smaller and consists primarily of RNA and a protein coat. The incubation period of hepatitis A is short, usually two to six weeks from contact with the virus. The virus presumably enters the liver from the intestine by way of the circulatory system. Large quantities of the virus can be present in the feces two to three weeks before the patient has any clinical symptoms, remaining an additional two weeks after symptoms begin. Most patients are no longer infectious to others three weeks after the onset of hepatitis-A symptoms. Unlike hepatitis B, a chronic carrier state for hepatitis-A virus in the stool or the blood is not thought to occur. The virus is apparently cleared from the body when the liver is healed.

Hepatitis B

Hepatitis B is also known as serum hepatitis or long-incubation hepatitis. The hepatitis-B virus differs from hepatitis A in that it is larger and contains DNA rather than RNA. This infection also has a different pattern of transmission. Hepatitis-B virus is not known to be present in the feces. Although some transmission of hepatitis B may occur from the ingestion of extremely large amounts of this virus under experimental conditions, hepatitis B is normally inactivated by the enzymes in the intestine; if hepatitis B is transmitted orally, the virus most likely enters the bloodstream through mucosal breaks in the mouth or the digestive tract above the intestine.

Hepatitis B has traditionally been associated with inoculation of blood or blood products through the skin. For example, hepatitis B is known to be spread by the use of shared needles by drug abusers, as well as by poorly steril-ized needles, dental equipment, ear-piercing devices, and even tattooing needles. Most cases of hepatitis transmitted by these means have disappeared with the use of disposable syringes and needles. Hepatitis B is still potentially transmitted via transfusions of immune serum and blood or plasma products. However, transmission of hepatitis B via these products or procedures has dramatically decreased because of the availability of markers that allow the detection of hepatitis-B particles in blood. Today hepatitis B is rarely, if ever, transmitted by blood transfusions.

On the other hand, hepatitis-B virus is present in the saliva, semen, vaginal secretions, and blood of infected people or carriers. Hepatitis-B virus is known to result in an asymptomatic carrier state in about 5 percent of infected people. This can be discovered only by a positive blood test for hepatitis-B surface antigen and does not necessarily imply the presence of chronic liver disease. A person may become a chronic carrier of hepatitis B without ever having had a recognizable case of active hepatitis, although, of course, a person may also become a carrier following a case of symptomatic hepatitis B.

Hepatitis B can be transmitted during vaginal intercourse if infected semen penetrates the vaginal mucosa. Transmission, however, depends both on the concentration of the virus in the semen and on the presence of microscopic bleeding points in the vagina (see below) that may occur during particularly heavy intercourse. Similarly, infected vaginal secretions, especially during and shortly after menstruation, also can penetrate the urethra or penis, presuming it has microscopic tears. These tiny bleeding points allow transmission of the virus to the bloodstream.

It is generally believed that transmission of hepatitis B

involves some contact with blood. The friction that occurs during vigorous vaginal or anal intercourse can produce microscopic abrasions, or small tears, in the tissues lining the vagina, the rectum, or even the penis. Microscopic bleeding points can also occur in the mouth as a result of brushing the teeth or even chewing food. These sites, not visible to the eye, might allow for transmission of hepatitis-B virus in either direction.

Hepatitis B can easily be transmitted by anal intercourse. During rectal intercourse bleeding points can develop in the lining of the rectum as a result of the trauma associated with repeated penetration. Semen or saliva containing hepatitis-B virus can then enter the bloodstream of the passive partner through these bleeding points. Conversely, blood containing hepatitis-B virus in the passive partner can infect the urethra or microscopic tears in the penis of the active partner.

Results of a recent study show that homosexual men are at an increased risk of contracting hepatitis-B infection if they have frequent sexual contact with multiple partners and practice active or passive anal intercourse, fist fornication, or active oral–anal sex. Rectal douching prior to intercourse also appears to increase the risk of hepatitis-B infection. Although used to cleanse the rectum prior to sex, vigorous douching can produce small bleeding points that will allow transmission of the virus.

Results also show that oral contact—kissing and fellatio with or without ejaculation—is not significantly associated with an increased risk of hepatitis-B infection. However, even though hepatitis-B virus is not carried or excreted in the feces, rectal bleeding may allow the presence of this virus in the rectum. Therefore, oral–anal contact with infected individuals may transmit the hepatitis-B virus from the rectum to the mouth, presumably through tiny mucosal irritations, or tears, on the tongue or by transmission across the oral mucous membranes. Also during oral sex, saliva containing viral particles may coat the penis, which may, in turn, infect a second partner during anal intercourse.

The presence of hepatitis-B infection is extremely common in homosexually active men. Approximately 6 percent of homosexual men attending STD clinics have evidence of this virus in their blood, and 55 to 60 percent of these men show some evidence of prior experience with hepatitis-B infections.

The major problem in controlling this infection is the fact that hepatitis B (as well as other forms of hepatitis) can cause infection without any symptoms. About two-thirds of hepatitis-B infections produce no obvious symptoms. Men and women who develop hepatitis-B infection without symptoms are, of course, at greater risk of unknowingly transmitting this infection to their sexual partners.

It is unlikely that simple kissing will result in the transmission of hepatitis B. However, since those infected with or carrying the virus have it present in the saliva, vigorous kissing could conceivably lead to the transmission of the virus in those cases in which kissing results in the exchange of saliva and when there are microscopic injuries to the tongue or to oral membranes. This is very difficult to study, and it has been impossible to prove that hepatitis B has been transmitted by kissing. However, in studies of hepatitis-B infections in homosexually active men, kissing has not been clearly associated with increased risk of infection. Thus, although it is possible to transmit hepatitis B by oral contact, the likelihood of this occurring is small. Hepatitis B can be transmitted among family members from parent to child (or vice versa) and from child to sibling. The exact mechanism of transmission is unclear, but kissing and the sharing of food, eating utensils, and toothbrushes may be involved.

A thorough description of hepatitis B can be useful in understanding the nature of this infection and the risks involved in transmitting this disease. The infectious hepatitis-B virus is known as the Dane particle, which consists of a core and a surface coat. Excess coating material shed by the virus can be found in the liver cells and blood serum of infected people.

Several components of the hepatitis virus, known as antigens, can be detected by immunological techniques. The hepatitis surface antigen (HBsAg) can be found in the coat of the Dane particle and in the excess coating material in the serum. People who have active hepatitis-B infection or who are carriers of this virus will have HBsAg detectable in their blood, and to a lesser degree in their saliva, semen, or vaginal secretions. HBsAg appears in the serum two to eight weeks after inoculation, depending on the location of viral entry. In most patients infected with hepatitis-B virus, HBsAg disappears from the serum and other body fluids six to eight weeks after the onset of symptoms, or four to five months after the original inoculation. About 5 to 10 percent of those infected with hepatitis-B virus remain chronic carriers of HBsAg and are therefore potentially infectious to others for an indeterminate period.

Antibodies to HBsAg (anti-HBs) begin to appear between several weeks and a few months after HBsAg has appeared. Antibodies to HBsAg can persist indefinitely, which implies protection against subsequent infection with the same subtype of hepatitis-B virus, but repeat episodes of hepatitis B with differing subtypes can occur. Hepatitis-B core antigen (HBcAg) is not usually detected in the serum, but antibodies to HBcAg (anti-HBc) are present very early in the course of the illness.

Another antigen, or component, of the hepatitis-B virus core is the e antigen. This antigen is present in the serum very early in the course of the infection, and when present it implies that the secretions of this patient are quite infectious. HBeAg remains in the serum for two to four months and begins to disappear when antibodies to HBeAg (anti-HBe) appear, implying a decrease in infectivity of the secretions.

Non-A Non-B Hepatitis

Another form of viral hepatitis has been described in the past several years. Until very recently the virus or viruses responsible for this form of hepatitis had not been identified. This form of hepatitis is not due to the hepatitis-A virus or the hepatitis-B virus, and is therefore known as non-A non-B hepatitis. It is likely that more than one virus is responsible for this form of hepatitis, because the symptoms of this disease are quite variable.

A virus has recently been isolated in cultured chimpanzee liver cells inoculated with plasma from a patient with non-A non-B hepatitis. This virus is larger than that of hepatitis A and hepatitis B, and may soon be renamed hepatitis-C virus.

Although there is evidence that non-A non-B hepatitis may be spread by sexual contact and contaminated needles, food, or water, the most frequent route of infection is through transfusion of contaminated blood or blood products, including some gamma globulin. Today most cases of transfusion-related hepatitis in the United States are due to non-A non-B hepatitis virus.

At present there is no blood test available for diagnosis of non-A non-B hepatitis, but with the identification of one of these viruses it is likely that this will be feasible soon. Currently, a patient with obvious hepatitis is diagnosed as having non-A non-B hepatitis if hepatitis A and B are ruled out.

SYMPTOMS

The symptoms produced by all of the different hepatitis viruses are relatively similar, although the incubation periods are different. Hepatitis-A symptoms develop in two to six weeks after exposure; hepatitis-B, one to four months; and non-A non-B, one to three months. Abnormalities in the functioning of the liver can be detected by laboratory tests prior to the development of any symptoms.

The course of viral hepatitis is extremely variable, and the majority of those infected develop no obvious symptoms. When symptoms do occur, they may include fatigue, sleeplessness, loss of appetite, and nausea. Low-grade fever and diarrhea may occur. Some people may notice a dull aching pain over the liver in the right upper part of the abdomen. Hepatitis B may occasionally produce pain in the joints and actual arthritis. Any of these symptoms may be present five to ten days before jaundice begins.

Jaundice is a yellowing of the skin, the eyes, and mucous membranes due to the presence of larger than usual amounts of bilirubin in the blood serum. Hepatitis damages liver cells, making it difficult for the liver to dispose of this excess bilirubin. The urine may become darker, and the stool much lighter. As jaundice becomes more advanced, most patients will begin to feel better, and the appetite will improve. Jaundice may last for as long as two or three weeks. Liver enzyme tests usually become almost normal by the time jaundice disappears.

The vast majority of people with hepatitis recover completely and without any long-term effects. But during the illness patients may feel a great deal of fatigue and may be unable to participate in their usual activities for as long as three to six months. Some people with active hepatitis B (less than 10 percent) become chronic carriers. About 5 percent of people infected with hepatitis-B virus may develop chronic active hepatitis, which may result in cirrhosis. Hepatitis B is also associated with one form of cancer of the liver, but the additional risk factors are not yet clearly known.

DIAGNOSIS

Diagnosis of hepatitis is usually suspected when typical signs and symptoms appear, including loss of appetite, dark urine, or jaundice. Laboratory tests of blood samples may reveal an increase in liver enzymes, as well as an increase of bilirubin in the blood serum. In addition, serum protein levels may be reduced. Blood serum may be examined for the presence of the antigen HBsAg or the antibody anti-HBc (see above). High levels of the antibody to hepatitis-A or -B virus indicate the recent presence of the virus. Diagnosis of non-A non-B hepatitis is made when blood tests rule out hepatitis-A or -B infection. Diagnosis of hepatitis is rarely made by a liver biopsy, although in some clinical situations (as with drug-induced hepatitis or tuberculosis) it may be necessary.

TREATMENT

There is little treatment for acute hepatitis, other than bed rest. Patients are not usually hospitalized for any of the three types of hepatitis except in very severe cases. Bed rest at home (rarely required for more than ten to fourteen days) is usually indicated because the patient's level of activity is restricted by his or her own level of energy. Hepatitis patients are usually advised to limit their activity to a level at which they feel comfortable. Mild exercise or activity does not appear to worsen the condition. Obviously, sexual activity should be prohibited during any phase of hepatitis, because of the risk of transmission to sexual partners. Alcohol and many medications should be limited during hepatitis, because these are metabolized or excreted by the liver. It is important for those with hepatitis to maintain a sufficient caloric intake even though the appetite may be depressed. Specific foods are not required or prohibited, but some people may have difficulty digesting fatty foods during hepatitis convalescence.

PREVENTION

Avoiding sexual contact with people known to be carriers of hepatitis-B virus and avoiding oral–anal contact with people known to be carrying hepatitis-A virus will minimize the risk of contracting this disease. Using a condom during vaginal or rectal intercourse may also limit the spread of hepatitis-B virus via these routes. People who do not have evidence of previous infection with hepatitis B (that is, those whose serum does not contain the antibody to the antigen HBsAg) can be protected against hepatitis-B infection by means of the new hepatitis-B vaccine, Heptavax. This vaccine is more than 90 percent effective and will minimize or eliminate the danger of hepatitis B in people at high risk, including homosexually active men and those health workers who are in frequent contact with blood serum.

Heptavax is prepared from the plasma of people who are carriers of the antigen HBsAg. This antigen is concentrated from the blood of these donors and is treated extensively to render these particles noninfectious. Because many of these donors are homosexually active men, there has been some concern about the possibility of contracting the acquired immunodeficiency syndrome from the vaccine. To date, however, there have been no cases of AIDS that are clearly related only to the use of this vaccine. The AIDS virus (HTLV-III, LAV), furthermore, is inactivated by the process used to prepare this vaccine. Currently being tested is a new genetically engineered hepatitis-B vaccine that would presumably remove any risk of contracting any other infectious disease from the vaccine.

A vaccine for hepatitis A is currently under investigation. Although one virus responsible for non-A non-B hepatitis has been discovered, as yet there is no vaccine available for this disease.

Gamma globulin (immune serum globulin) has been used in intramuscular injections to prevent hepatitis from developing in those exposed to the hepatitis-A virus. It has been quite effective in preventing or ameliorating the infection in those likely to come into contact with hepatitis A. Specific hyperimmune serum against hepatitis B—hepatitis-B immune globulin (HBIG)—is available but extremely expensive. If it is administered within forty-eight hours after contamination with hepatitis B, HBIG is effective in preventing or ameliorating infection due to this virus. The effectiveness of these products in preventing non-A non-B hepatitis following exposure is not clearly known.

Hepatitis-A virus is not thought to cross the placenta or be found in breast milk. Hepatitis B, however, can possibly be transmitted from mother to infant at the time of delivery. Infants born of antigen-positive mothers should receive the vaccine plus HBIG. This will prevent the carrier state from developing in the infant and will decrease the risk of liver cancer later in life. Infants of these mothers rarely develop symptomatic hepatitis, however. Mothers who are HBsAg carriers can transmit this virus either from breast milk or from the small amounts of blood that may contaminate cracked nipples early in nursing.

8 / Sexually Transmitted Diseases in Homosexuals

The last fifteen to twenty years have seen a dramatic increase in the awareness of sexually transmitted infections in homosexuals. Most of these infections appear to be borne by homosexually active men. Much less is known about sexually transmitted diseases in homosexually active women.

Lesbians have considerably lower rates of the more common sexually transmitted diseases than do heterosexually active women, and these rates are certainly much lower than those in gay men. Lesbians may have a slightly increased risk of transmitting hepatitis A and certain types of vaginitis caused by yeastlike fungi and trichomoniasis. These lower rates in lesbians are probably attributable to a much lower number of different sexual contacts. Shared towels and vaginal-douching equipment may be associated with some sexually transmitted infections in lesbian women.

Sexually transmitted infections in gay men, on the other hand, have reached epidemic proportions. Aside from AIDS, which is discussed in the next chapter, an ever-increasing list of infections has been noted in the past decade. Until recently, many physicians have not been aware of the nature of sexual practices among gay men. This unawareness, along with the fear of exposure of sexual identity and the anticipation of rejection, has prevented many gay men from receiving appropriate and thorough medical care.

For the above reasons it has been difficult to determine the risk factors associated with specific sexually transmitted infections in gay men. The "risk factor" is a procedure, an activity, an event, or an associated condition that is predictive of a higher likelihood of disease. Risk factors for such cardiovascular diseases as heart attacks and strokes have been identified relatively easily and include obesity, increased cholesterol, cigarette smoking, and high blood pressure. The usefulness of determining risk factors for diseases is that once they are identified, a modification in these factors is usually, but not always, associated with a decreased risk of acquiring the particular disease.

Why are gay men so susceptible to sexually transmitted infections? There is nothing about homosexuality per se that predisposes one to an increased rate of infection. Sexual acts performed by gay men in and of themselves do not result in infection when performed with a single partner. Many, if not most, of the sexual activities performed by gay men are performed by heterosexual couples as well. However, in one segment of the gay population, multiple sexual contacts with a large number of different individuals are quite common under conditions that often preserve anonymity and preclude bathing, cleansing, and other preventive measures. Under these conditions, it is impossible to know the previous sexual health histories of one's partners, and it is relatively easy to understand how, once introduced, any infectious agent can spread rapidly.

Gay couples may not be exclusively monogamous. Long-term gay relationships may be punctuated with outside sexual relations. Information about sexually transmitted diseases to which gay men are prone has only recently been widely disseminated among these high-risk individuals.

Not all homosexually active men are at equal risk of developing sexually transmitted diseases. The overwhelming majority of medical studies dealing with sexual practices and STDs in gay men are derived from data collected in public clinics that provide health care to people generally living in large cities. Those who attend these STD clinics may differ significantly from those who receive their medical care from private or other sources. Despite the abundance of information available from public clinics, none is totally relevant regarding the sexual practices and the incidence of STDs in gay men in general. Monogamous homosexual couples and lifetime partners are at no greater risk of contracting an STD than are similar heterosexually active couples.

Certain STDs are more likely to occur in homosexually active men than in heterosexuals. Based on information again derived from public STD clinics, studies show that gonorrhea, the early stages of syphilis, and anal-rectal warts are more frequent among gay men, while nongonococcal urethritis, herpes, and genital warts are more common in heterosexual men. Hepatitis B is also seen more frequently in gay men than in straight men. These diseases are discussed in detail in other chapters.

In addition to gonorrhea, syphilis, and anal-rectal warts, gay men with multiple sexual partners are also susceptible to hepatitis A and B, genital and anal-rectal herpes, crab louse infestations, cytomegalovirus infections, urethral and anal-rectal infections with meningococci (cousins of the gonorrhea bacterium), and a variety of bacterial, viral, and parasitic infections or infestations of the gastrointestinal tract. These latter diseases will be discussed in detail in this chapter.

Gastrointestinal infections or infestations are quite common in gay men and have been referred to as the "gay bowel syndrome." The use of the term "syndrome" is really not appropriate, as it implies some common underlying cause. A variety of different symptoms may occur and may be caused by the presence of one or more infecting organisms that are sexually transmissible. Many of these organisms, however, may not produce any symptoms of intestinal distress. Thus the person without symptoms may be just as contagious as the person with mild diarrhea or abdominal distress. Different organisms may produce similar symptoms, and more than one organism may be present simultaneously.

The specific health needs of homosexually active men have been recognized by the medical profession only recently. The increase in sexual freedom that has been associated with the broadening STD epidemic in the past two decades has brought many gay men face to face with health-care providers who may, or may not, understand their sexuality.

Thus, the STD patient who conceals his homosexuality may place himself in double jeopardy in many cases by pre-

venting well-meaning physicians from evaluating or pur-
suing certain diseases that are now well known to be
sexually transmitted. The epidemic of AIDS in homosexually
active men has particularly helped to underscore both the
health needs of the gay patient and the requisite awareness
and openness of the medical profession. It is hoped that
physicians will become more understanding of the sexual
needs of gay patients and that, in turn, gay patients will
become more open and direct with their physicians about
their sexual orientation.

Sexually Transmitted Bowel Infections

Gay sexual activity may result in contracting disease-
causing pathogens at either end of the gastrointestinal
tract, which begins at the mouth and ends at the anus.
Organisms may be introduced orally through oral–genital
or oral–anal contact. Similarly, organisms may be introduced anally through anal intercourse, fist fornication, or
finger insertion.

The intestinal diseases usually found in homosexual men
also occur as nonsexually transmitted diseases. For example,
shigellosis, amebic dysentery, and giardiasis commonly
occur as food-borne or water-borne outbreaks in a variety
of locations around the world. The past ten years have seen
a dramatic increase in the occurrence of these gastrointestinal disorders in people who either lack a history of
foreign travel or have no link to a food- or water-borne
outbreak. Most of these latter patients turn out to be homosexually active men.

The astounding increase in cases of parasitic and bacterial bowel infections may have resulted from the fact that these organisms may be present in the bowel of gay men without necessarily producing symptoms. Therefore, an unassuming, otherwise healthy person who is carrying amoeba, giardia, or shigella organisms may pass them to his sexual partners without knowing that he himself is affected. Oral–anal sex is not the only means by which these organisms can spread. Oral–genital sex with a person who has recently been involved in anal intercourse may transmit a small number of these organisms from the penis to the active partner's mouth and subsequently to the gastrointestinal tract.

Although rectal douching (enemas) is usually thought to be a cleansing mechanism, it may in fact wash some parasites into the rectal area. Small numbers of these organisms may be quite infectious and spread to the penis or the scrotum after a bowel movement or an enema. These organisms may then be transmitted to the mouth from the penis or the scrotal areas.

Many of these organisms have become hyperendemic in the gay communities of large cities in the United States. An endemic infection is one that tends to occur in a limited segment of a given population. A hyperendemic infection is one in which an infecting organism is present in a large percent of the particular segment. Not every infected person becomes clinically ill, but the agents are nevertheless present in a large proportion of the community. Many parasites and intestinal pathogens have become hyperendemic because they are frequently passed among gay males who have a large number of anonymous sexual contacts.

Most of the diseases discussed below are spread by oral–anal contact or by anal–genital intercourse. Prevention of gastrointestinal infections can be achieved by limiting oral–anal contact to a single partner who is known to be monogamous and free of the parasites and bacteria mentioned; by using a condom during anal intercourse; and by limiting the number of sexual contacts, and avoiding anonymous sexual encounters in which the health status of the sexual partner is not known.

Proctitis

Proctitis is inflammation of the rectum. It may result from infection due to a variety of infectious organisms or from trauma caused by the insertion of large objects, including the hand or the fist, into the rectum during sexual stimulation. Proctitis may also occur as noninfectious inflammatory bowel disease such as ulcerative colitis. Not all types of proctitis are sexually transmitted; however, this discussion will be limited to those that are.

The symptoms associated with proctitis include pain and fullness and itching around the anus or the rectum. Pain or difficulty during bowel movements may be experienced, and a puslike discharge may also be present. Some patients notice pus or blood in their stool or staining on their underwear. Although constipation is somewhat more frequent, diarrhea is also sometimes experienced. Some or all of the symptoms may be present at any one time. In general, the symptoms per se do not imply the presence of one or another specific cause, and, in fact, many patients with proctitis may have more than one organism responsible for their symptoms. All of the organisms that are responsible for this disease can be found in approximately 40 percent of gay men attending STD clinics who do not report any symptoms of proctitis.

Proctitis may be due to the presence of *Neisseria gonorrhoeae*, the organism of gonorrhea, or *Neisseria meningitidis*, an organism of meningitis. Anal gonorrhea may produce a puslike discharge, and diagnosis is made by culturing pus obtained by a rectal swab. Usually your physician will obtain a specimen prior to examination of the rectal mucosa with an anoscope, which must be lubricated to allow for easy insertion. Many of these lubricants inhibit the growth of some bacteria; therefore, appropriate cultures should be taken before the instrument is inserted.

Anal gonorrhea can be effectively treated with various antibiotics.

Proctitis may also be caused by herpes simplex virus, and symptoms may include severe rectal or anal pain, numbness or tingling in the area around the anus or in the thighs, fever, and swelling of the glands in the groin. Some men may have difficulty passing urine during an acute attack of herpes-induced proctitis. As with other herpes infections, the first attack is usually the most severe, with recurrences being somewhat milder. Diagnosis is made by inspection and culture of typical herpes in the anal area or ulcers in the rectal area with an anoscope.

Most episodes of herpes proctitis will resolve spontaneously with sitz baths and pain medication, but the new drug acyclovir is currently being evaluated for the treatment of this condition.

The organism that causes nongonococcal urethritis,

Chlamydia trachomatis, may also cause nongonococcal proctitis. The strain of chlamydia that causes lymphogranuloma venereum (see Chapter 10) may also cause specific proctitis with ulcers in or around the rectum. Antibiotics can be used to treat proctitis due to chlamydia.

Syphilis may also occur in the anal or rectal area with or without symptoms. The primary chancre may occur in this area without the typical appearance it has on the external genitals. A chancre deep within the rectum can be seen only with an anoscope. Diagnosis of syphilis in this area is made by microscopic examination of material obtained from a typical ulcer and/or by blood test. Syphilis in this area is treated with penicillin or other antibiotics.

Anal warts may also produce symptoms of proctitis and may be present with any of the other causes of this condition.

Trauma-induced infection, particularly caused by heavy rectal intercourse or fist/object insertion, may produce microscopic tears in the rectal mucosa, as well as fissures or tears in the anal area. Sometimes these traumatic tears, or tiny bleeding points, become infected with organisms normally present in the stool.

Other Intestinal Problems: Enteritis, Colitis, and Proctocolitis

The area of the intestine that is infected in a particular case is often difficult to determine, but, in general, as the upper portions of the bowel are involved, different symptoms may occur. Patients with enteritis (inflammation of the intestine) have loose, watery stools, fever, chills, achiness, and abdominal cramps. Some enteric infections cause an increase in flatulence, bloating, upper-abdominal discomfort or pain, and a variety of abnormal stools, including bloody or flaky stools. Milder forms of enteritis may simply produce increased frequency of stools with mild abdominal cramps.

Shigellosis is one of the most frequent enteric diseases among gay men. The shigella organism can be transmitted by a relatively small number of live bacteria. This disease can be quite severe with watery diarrhea, abdominal cramping, high fever, and chills. Blood or mucus may be present in the stools. Diagnosis is made by culturing the shigella organism from the stool. Although many patients may spontaneously recover without antibiotics, some doctors prescribe them routinely. It is important for anyone recovering from shigellosis to refrain from sexual activity until his stool cultures have been rendered negative, either with specific treatment or with the passage of time.

Other bacteria have been implicated as sexually transmitted causes of bowel infection. These include campylobacter, an organism frequently responsible for community outbreaks of diarrhea, and salmonella, a bacteria also associated with outbreaks of gastroenteritis. A few people have developed typhoid fever as a result of sexual transmission. Typhoid fever is caused by a special strain of salmonella.

Most physicians will not treat salmonella or campylobacter gastroenteritis, because treatment may simply prolong the asymptomatic or carrier state and might potentially cause increased resistance among these infecting organisms. Typhoid fever, on the other hand, is always treated and generally responds to appropriate antibiotics. Some physicians may choose to treat campylobacter diarrhea, which might shorten the symptomatic period.

Colitis (inflammation of the large intestine) may be caused by the parasitic amoeba *Entamoeba histolytica*. This parasite is the cause of amebic dysentery, and outbreaks of this disease occur all over the world. In large American cities, however, most people with amoebic infestations who do not have a history of foreign travel are gay men. Amoebas may be present as cysts in the stools of nonsymptomatic patients and may be passed by oral–anal sex to partners who may, in turn, develop symptomatic disease.

Amebiasis is usually associated with bloating, mild or vague pain in the abdomen, and constipation or diarrhea. Some patients have symptoms limited to the rectum which may appear as proctitis alone (see above). In many cases the symptoms are quite mild and may come and go over several months. This pattern may prevent infected people from receiving appropriate diagnosis and therapy, which may thereby increase the spread of this infestation to sexual contacts during this period.

Amebiasis is diagnosed by identifying the amoeba in the stool or in the ulcerative lesions of the rectum seen through an anoscope. Several stool specimens may have to be examined in order to find this organism. There is an available new test—which may soon become the standard—that can detect small amounts of amoebic antigens in the stool. Very rarely, gay patients with amoebic infestations may develop liver abscesses, but in general this disease is limited to the intestinal tract.

Most physicians will treat intestinal amebiasis with

metronidazole (Flagyl) or dilozanide (Entamide or Furamide). Many other drugs may also be used, such as paromomycin (Humatin) or tetracycline. Patients with no symptoms, but whose stool contains amoebic cysts, are usually treated with diloxanide or iodoquinol (Diodoquin) with or without tetracycline.

Giardiasis is an enteric infestation of the protozoan parasite *Giardia lamblia*. This infestation generally involves the upper portion of the small intestine and produces symptoms of watery diarrhea, bloating, nausea, abdominal pain or distress, flatulence, and loss of appetite. This organism may be present for many months without producing symptoms. Generally when symptoms occur they develop at least a week or ten days after exposure. This disease often occurs in combination with amebiasis. Oral–anal sex and oral–genital sex are usually responsible for transmission of the organism in homosexual men. Giardiasis may also develop as a result of drinking water contaminated with the parasite, although this is relatively uncommon in the United States.

Diagnosis is not always possible by stool-specimen examination, as the organism is passed only infrequently into the feces. However, a string may be swallowed, withdrawn, and then examined microscopically for the giardia organism, which is often found in the upper duodenum. In some cases a duodenal biopsy may be necessary. Treatment is generally successful and involves the use of quinacrine (Atabrine) or metronidazole (Flagyl). Oral–anal sex should be avoided until a repeat string test is negative for this organism.

Sexually related infections can also be caused by worms

that may be transmitted through oral–anal sex. A frequent sexually transmitted worm is the pinworm or threadworm (*Enterobius vermicularis*), and the most common symptom associated with this organism is intense itching around the anus, especially at night. The worms leave the rectum at night and lay their eggs in the area of the external anus. The Scotch Tape test, whereby tape is placed over the anus during the night and then sent for microscopic examination the next morning, can reveal the presence of these eggs. Sexual partners should be examined and treated appropriately with Antiminth or Vermox.

Several reports have suggested that homosexual men participating in anal-receptive intercourse for several years may be at an increased risk of developing cancer of the anus, but the precise reason is unclear. Prevention of these and other diseases is discussed more fully in Chapter 11.

9 / Acquired Immunodeficiency Syndrome (AIDS)

No disease has received so much press and inspired so much concern among doctors and the public alike in recent years as the acquired immunodeficiency syndrome (AIDS). The acquired immunodeficiency syndrome was unknown to medical investigators until 1980, when a few clustered cases of Kaposi's sarcoma, and also those of *Pneumocystis carinii* pneumonia (PCP), appeared in otherwise healthy men. Kaposi's sarcoma, a fleshy tumor of blood vessels in the skin and other organs, was previously seen in elderly men. *Pneumocystis carinii* pneumonia, an opportunistic infection (one that takes advantage of an immunosuppressed host) caused by a presumed protozoan parasite, is a life-threatening progressive lung disease that usually occurs in patients with defective immunity such as that caused by leukemia and certain other cancers, including lymphomas and Hodgkin's disease.

These reports of the occurrence of Kaposi's sarcoma and *Pneumocystis carinii* pneumonia in previously healthy young men with no known immune defects were first made public in June 1981. At that time thirty-one cases were reported: five cases of *Pneumocystis carinii* and twenty-six cases of both Kaposi's sarcoma and PCP. The patients all lived in Los Angeles or New York City and were either homosexually active men and/or intravenous drug abusers.

Detailed medical and laboratory studies indicated that these patients had acquired a defect in their cellular immune system. Normal immunity to infections (and probably to cancer) is comprised of two cooperating systems: the *humoral* and *cellular* immune systems. The humoral immune system is responsible for the production of antibodies, which protect against infection by several means. These antibodies are necessary, for example, to prepare certain kinds of bacteria for ingestion by active white blood cells or phagocytes. Antibodies are produced when stimulated by antigens—certain components of bacteria, viruses, and other infecting agents. Specialized cells responsible for the production of antibodies include B-lymphocytes, plasma cells, and macrophages. The humoral immune system in patients with AIDS was once thought to be normal, but recent evidence suggests that B-lymphocytes may not respond normally to certain new stimulants, and in fact there may be overstimulation of the antibody-producing mechanism, resulting in new antigens that may not elicit the appropriate immune response.

The cellular immune system is responsible for cell-mediated immunity. It provides defense against infection due to viruses, fungi, the organisms of tuberculosis, certain kinds of bacteria that act intracellularly, and some protozoal infections, primarily those caused by *Pneumocystis carinii*,

cryptosporidia, and *Toxoplasma gondii.* The cellular immune system is also responsible for the rejection of grafts
of foreign tissue and is thought to play an important role
in the immune surveillance against tumors. This latter
mechanism may be an important defense against the
development of some cancers. Cellular immunity is primarily mediated by the T-lymphocyte, a cell that secretes
immune-active substances called lymphokines. There are
several different subsets of T-lymphocytes, most notably
the helper, or inducer, T-cells and the suppressor, or cyto-
toxic, T-cells. Patients with AIDS have a decreased number
of helper T-cells and a decreased ratio of helper to suppressor T-cells.

In the forty-eight months since the initial cases were reported, more than eight thousand patients with AIDS have
been documented and reported to the Centers for Disease
Control (CDC). About one hundred new cases are reported each week, and until recently the number of new
cases has been doubling every six months. The number of
new AIDS cases reported continues to rise, although the
rate of increase may be slowing down.

Certain individuals are at an increased risk of developing
AIDS, but all of the risk factors associated with this disease
are not yet known. Although the cause of AIDS has
recently been determined, the specific types of sexual
activity responsible for its transmission have not been completely documented. Nonetheless, epidemiological studies
have provided a general picture of the disease and allow
us to determine those who are at the greatest risk.

Approximately 71 percent of the reported cases of AIDS
are homosexually or bisexually active men between the ages

of twenty and forty-five. Most, but not all, of the homosexual men with AIDS have had a large number of sexual partners. One report found that gay men with AIDS averaged eleven hundred different sexual partners in a lifetime, compared to similar groups of gay men without AIDS who averaged about five hundred lifetime sexual partners. Thus, a large number of sexual partners clearly increases the risk of AIDS.

Although the exact transmission route of the AIDS-associated virus by sexual means is not known, more patients with AIDS practiced oral–anal contact and fist fornication than did a comparable group of gay men without AIDS. However, these sexual activities are not practiced by all patients who have developed AIDS. Receptive anal intercourse may also be a risk factor. The AIDS patients had a higher number of male sexual partners per year and were more likely to have had sex in bathhouses than the non-AIDS group. It is not known whether AIDS can be transmitted by intimate kissing or by fellatio (with or without the swallowing of semen). However, the AIDS-associated virus is present in saliva, semen, and blood of infected patients.

Contamination with blood or blood products seems to be an important risk factor in the development of AIDS. The occurrence of AIDS in the population tends to mimic that of hepatitis B in that it is transmissible both sexually and parenterally (by administration of blood or blood products or by needle). Intravenous drug abusers are therefore at a higher risk of contracting AIDS, with approximately 20 percent of AIDS patients being in this category. Presumably the AIDS-associated virus is transmitted from person to person by means of contaminated needles used for injection.

The occurrence of AIDS in heterosexual hemophiliac men who have received lifelong transfusions of blood or plasma components, necessary to control the tendency of these people to bleed, further confirms the transmissibility of the AIDS-associated virus via the blood. Patients with hemophilia may receive a clotting factor of plasma made either from single, few, or multiple donors. The product concentrated from the blood of multiple donors may be derived from as many as two or three thousand individual donors. Hemophiliac patients require several transfusions of this material weekly or monthly, and the possibilities of dissemination of the AIDS-associated virus in this way are enormous.

The risk of acquiring AIDS from a single- or multiple-unit transfusion of blood during surgery or in other clinical situations requiring blood is not known, but it is probably extremely low. AIDS is known to have been transmitted to blood recipients from donors who were themselves healthy nonsymptomatic carriers of the AIDS-associated virus at the time of their blood donation, many of whom remain healthy. This is important evidence of the existence of a carrier state for this virus in high-risk people with no obvious clinical disease.

The recent identification of a specific virus associated with AIDS and the development of a blood test for antibodies to this agent now make it possible to screen donated blood and eliminate blood transfusions as a risk for this illness. Currently, however, people in high-risk groups (homosexual men with many partners, intravenous drug abusers, Haitians) are advised to voluntarily refrain from donating blood. There is no danger of contracting AIDS while donating blood.

There is no evidence that AIDS can be spread by swimming pools, public toilets, restaurants, or any other public places. AIDS is not highly contagious and is not spread by casual contact. In fact, only about 5 to 20 percent of sexual partners of patients with AIDS have themselves developed the syndrome, although these results are still early.

In addition to those already mentioned, AIDS has been reported in a small number of women who have been sexual contacts of men with known or presumed AIDS or men at risk of contracting AIDS by means of their sexual habits or intravenous drug use. AIDS has also been reported in several children of mothers who abuse drugs. It is possible that the virus passes through the placenta during the developmental stages of pregnancy. It is also possible, but has not in any way been proved, that close contact between the high-risk mother and her child may also somehow allow the transmission of this disease. AIDS has also been reported in heterosexual female prostitutes.

Another group identified with AIDS are recent immigrants of both sexes from Haiti in such metropolitan areas as Miami and New York City. Most of these patients are alleged to be heterosexual and do not admit to the use of intravenous drugs. Although health records are not optimal, the occurrence of AIDS is well known in Haiti, with more than 120 cases reported. This syndrome was not seen before 1979, as in the United States. About 30 to 50 percent of these patients do not have any of the other known risk factors.

AIDS is also occurring in alarming numbers in central Africa, especially in Zaire and neighboring countries. Although more than ten thousand cases are believed to have been diagnosed in Zaire, none probably existed ten or more years ago. These individuals are not necessarily homosexual, with both men and women having been affected equally. It is possible that AIDS originated in Africa and then spread to Haiti after a large number of Haitian workers migrated to Africa about a decade ago and later returned to Haiti. How AIDS was initially transmitted to American homosexual men or drug users is also unclear, but it may have been introduced by Haitian men carrying the AIDS-associated virus. There is also the possibility that American men introduced AIDS into Haiti, but proof for any of these hypotheses is lacking.

AIDS has been reported in France, Germany, Belgium, England, Holland, and many other European countries, although the number of cases in each country is much lower than in the United States. In these countries AIDS occurs in the same risk groups as in America.

AIDS has also occurred in prisons, but it is unclear whether drug abuse and homosexual activity have been eliminated as possible associated variables.

The major cause of AIDS has only recently been isolated. Researchers at the National Institutes of Health (NIH), in Bethesda, and the Institut Pasteur, in Paris, have isolated retroviruses from patients with AIDS and the AIDS-related complex (see below). Retroviruses are small RNA viruses that contain a reverse transcriptase enzyme that codes for the homologous viral DNA to be manufactured by the infected host cell. It seems likely that the French and American scientists have identified the same or a similar type of virus.

The AIDS-associated virus has been labeled by Dr. Robert

Gallo of the NIH as HTLV-III, for Human T-cell lymphotropic Virus III. The French researchers have named their virus LAV, for lymphadenopathy-associated virus. HTLV-I is a virus associated with T-cell leukemia, a rare blood disease found especially in southern Japan, possibly brought from Africa by Portuguese sailors in the sixteenth century. HTLV-II is a retrovirus associated with hairy-cell leukemia, another rare form of leukemia. More than 95 percent of tested patients with AIDS and AIDS-related complex have antibodies to HTLV-III in their blood serum, as do 30 to 65 percent of asymptomatic homosexual men in high-risk areas. Antibodies to LAV have been detected in 65 percent of nonsymptomatic homosexual men attending STD clinics in San Francisco and in about 50 percent of a similar group in New York City. More than 80 percent of heavy intravenous drug abusers in New York have antibodies to LAV. Dr. Luc Montagnier and his colleagues at the Institut Pasteur reported that 13 to 38 percent of AIDS patients and 9 to 75 percent of AIDS-related-complex patients (see below) had antibodies to LAV, depending on the method used to detect the antibody.

DIAGNOSIS

At present, AIDS is a complex of several signs and symptoms. Physicians can suspect this diagnosis when previously healthy individuals from the groups described above develop fever; weight loss; small, widely scattered fleshy purplish skin lesions consistent with Kaposi's sarcoma; and/or a variety of proven opportunistic infections (those usually found in seriously ill people with defective cellular immunity). These infections can present as pneumonia, meningitis, encephalitis, severe diarrhea, serious and difficult oral or vaginal thrush (monilia or candida infection), and/or herpes infection that extends beyond the usual locations on the genitalia or around the mouth. A variety of other infections may occur, including tuberculosis, atypical tuberculosis, and cryptosporidiosis.

An additional diagnostic problem is the indeterminate latency period of AIDS before symptoms become apparent. Certain epidemiological findings suggest that the latency period from presumed exposure to the AIDS-associated virus to the development of clinical illness may range from six months or less to as long as five years.

A syndrome known as AIDS-related complex (ARC) or lymphadenopathy syndrome has also been described with increasing frequency affecting homosexually active men and other high-risk groups. Up to 20 percent of gay men in certain areas of San Francisco have ARC. These patients may have fever, malaise, weight loss, night sweats, diarrhea, and nonspecific but widespread swelling of the lymph nodes in the neck, under the arms, in the groin, and elsewhere. These patients may spontaneously improve, while others may relapse at a later date. It is not known whether all of these patients will ultimately develop AIDS or whether they will be at risk of developing other infection; in some cities but not in others, up to 20 percent of patients with ARC have developed AIDS. Further studies are under way to fully define the ARC syndrome. Some researchers prefer the term "lymphadenopathy syndrome" to "ARC" because it is unclear whether ARC is ultimately related to AIDS.

Understandably, many of those in the high-risk groups

mentioned above are seriously concerned about the likeli-hood of their contracting AIDS. Some studies have shown that apparently healthy, sexually active homosexual men without any evidence of AIDS or ARC have a reduced ratio of T-helper to T-suppressor cells. Many common infections—transmitted sexually or otherwise—may in-crease T-suppressor cells and therefore lower the T-helper to T-suppressor ratio. This may be transient or permanent and may or may not be related to the risk of AIDS or the presence of HTLV-III or LAV. A depressed T-helper to T-suppressor ratio is not therefore diagnostic of AIDS.

TREATMENT

There is no known treatment for AIDS, although many of the associated infections can be treated and controlled. Patients may recover from these infections with appropriate intensive treatment, but ultimately many of them will develop additional life-threatening infections. Drugs such as ribavirin and suramin have in vitro activity against HTLV-III and clinical trials are in progress. Recombinant-derived gamma interferon and interleukin 2, products of normally functioning lymphocytes, are being studied and may ameliorate the cellular immune defects in some patients. These substances also may be used to treat some patients with Kaposi's sarcoma. Kaposi's sarcoma can also be treated with radiotherapy; some of these patients have been cured of the sarcoma. But the unfortunate nature of the immuno-deficiency syndrome is that patients with AIDS are subject to constant, multiple infections, some of which may not respond to therapy and may ultimately result in death. The mortality rate from the early diagnosed cases approaches

80 percent. Overall, approximately 45 percent of all diagnosed patients with AIDS have died.

Most states require that physicians report cases of AIDS to the health department. The purpose is to ascertain the numbers of cases for accurate statistics so that the Centers for Disease Control can continue their investigation. The reporting of AIDS cases is not used for contact-tracing disease control as with syphilis or gonorrhea. The names of individual patients are never released, and the highest degree of confidentiality is maintained.

Some states with many cases of AIDS also request that ARC cases be reported and studied. At least some of those patients with ARC do recover completely without developing AIDS.

Most patients with AIDS will be hospitalized at the time the diagnosis is confirmed. The severity of the infections that actually lead to a diagnosis of AIDS usually necessitates hospitalization for treatment. When the infection is successfully treated, most patients will return home, and many may return to work.

Most major cities with large gay communities have AIDS support groups, action committees, and/or clinics. These organizations can be helpful in answering questions about AIDS or ARC and relieving anxiety with professional counseling. The National Gay Task Force maintains an AIDS crisis telephone line at 1-800-221-7044.

PREVENTION

With the cause of AIDS having been identified only recently, and the method of transmission not yet fully documented, it is impossible to know how to prevent this disease. However, the risk of contracting AIDS can be minimized by avoiding sexual contact with patients with known or suspected AIDS. AIDS is not likely to be spread by casual contact, but transmission is most likely to involve exchange of such body fluids as blood, urine, semen, and possibly saliva. Homosexual men should decrease the number of their sexual contacts and eliminate anonymous sexual encounters if at all possible. Similarly, since the risk of AIDS in heterosexual men and women remains unknown, the number of casual sexual contacts should also be limited.

The Centers for Disease Control have recommended that all people at risk of developing AIDS refrain voluntarily from making blood donations. This would include recent Haitian immigrants, drug abusers, and homosexually or bisexually active men with multiple sexual partners. The identification of the AIDS-associated virus has rapidly led to the development of an antibody test that will be able to screen blood and eliminate at least one route of transmissibility of this disease. This blood test will be available in 1985, but additional studies will also be necessary to understand what a positive test means in an asymptomatic individual.

Although the HLTV-III/LAV antibody blood test is not available routinely, many gay health services are collecting bloods for this analysis. At the present time little is known about the implications of a positive antibody test in an asymptomatic homosexual man or in a drug abuser. Certainly, the presence of antibodies in the blood serum to HTLV-III/LAV represents previous exposure to or infection with the virus. However, a positive test may mean that the individual has handled the infection, has processed it normally, and will not become ill or develop outright AIDS. On the other hand, a positive test might imply that the individual is infected and may later become ill or may spread the infection to sexual partners.

It is hoped that these questions and others about immunity to infection with the AIDS-associated virus and the natural history of this infection will be answered in the course of the next few years as the result of ongoing studies.

Gay sexual activities that involve exchange of body fluids and/or blood contamination include anal intercourse and fist fornication. Mutual masturbation is not likely to be implicated in the spread of AIDS, and the risks associated with kissing and oral–genital sex cannot yet be accurately determined. To avoid increased susceptibility to disease, gay men and others at high risk should care for their general health and insure adequate nutrition, rest, sleep, and exercise.

10/ Other Sexually Transmitted Diseases

The list of "other" diseases that are thought to be transmitted sexually has grown considerably during the past several years. Many of these diseases used to be known as the minor sexually transmitted diseases. In my experience, however, all have been hardly "minor" to the patients who suffer from them. Some of these diseases are rarely seen in the United States (such as lymphogranuloma venereum or chancroid), but even these diseases have become more frequent in the past few years. Other diseases such as genital warts are extremely common and quite bothersome. Some of these diseases, including mononucleosis and molluscum contagiosum, may also be spread by other than sexual means, although close contact is usually required for their transmission.

Balanitis

"Balanitis" is a term given to infection of the glans, or head, of the penis. It may be due to a variety of infectious agents, including the agent of gonorrhea, trichomonads, streptococci, yeastlike fungi (such as candida), and the organism of syphilis. Many noninfectious causes of this condition exist and include psoriasis and other skin disorders.

The infectious organisms can be transmitted during sexual intercourse and are usually present in the vagina or rectum of the sexual partner. Diagnosis is made by inspection and culture. Identification of the organism and treatment with appropriate antibiotics or antifungal agents usually result in a cure. (See Gonorrhea, Chapter 1; Vaginitis and Cervicitis, Chapter 4; and Syphilis, Chapter 6.)

Bartholin's Gland Abscess

There are small glands in the vulva of a woman that drain through the labia minora. Normally these glands are hardly noticed, but they can become infected with bacteria. When this occurs there is painful swelling of the Bartholin's gland, and the labia may become swollen. Infection of these glands can occur with *E. coli*, Bacteroides species, *Neisseria gonorrhoeae*, and genital mycoplasmas. Similarly, there are small glands, known as Skene's glands, located near the female urethral opening. These can occasionally become infected with bacteria or with *Trichomonas vaginalis*. Pain on urination is experienced, and, on occasion, pus may be found at this site. Diagnosis is made by examination of the discharge from these glands, and treatment is directed at the causative organisms.

Sexual transmissibility and prevention of these infections remains poorly understood.

Chancroid

Chancroid is a sexually transmitted disease that produces ulcerations on the external genitalia that are similar to, but usually distinguishable from, the lesions of syphilis. Chancroid usually begins as small pimples, or papules, which appear within five to ten days of sexual contact with an infected person. This disease produces shallow, single or multiple ulcers, or sores, that are typically but not always painful, have ragged edges, and are generally soft. They may be covered with a whitish or grayish puslike material, and there may be tender enlargement of the lymph nodes in the groin. Lesions may be found on the head or the shaft of the penis, in the vagina, on the labia, or around the anus. These lesions in their early stages may be mistaken for genital herpes, and they must always be distinguished from syphilis. Occasionally chancroid will spread to the lymph nodes. Both sexes can be asymptomatic carriers. Chancroid most likely cannot be transmitted to a baby during pregnancy or while breast-feeding.

The cause of chancroid is believed to be a bacterium that is somewhat difficult to grow in the laboratory, but diagnosis is usually made by this means. Newer diagnostic tests for use in blood-serum analysis are being developed. Diagnosis of chancroid is made by examining material from the base of the ulcer to exclude the *Treponema pallidum* organism and the herpes simplex virus. If a swollen gland is present in the groin, aspiration of the pus from this gland is useful for culturing the causative agent of chancroid, *Hemophilus ducreyi*. Other organisms may be implicated in the cause of chancroid.

Previously chancroid was limited to Africa and Asia, but recent outbreaks in Winnipeg, Canada, and Orange County, California, have been described and attributed to frequent contact with infected prostitutes. Chancroid is now seen in New York City and elsewhere in the United States.

Chancroid is treated with antibiotics. A variety of drugs is effective, especially sulfa drugs alone or in combination with trimethoprim. Other antibiotics, including streptomycin, kanamycin, erythromycin, or the tetracyclines, are also effective. Early treatment of known contacts may prevent the ulceration. Condom use may prevent transmission, but this has not been proved. Chancroid is a reportable STD. It is best prevented by identification and treatment of those infected and those exposed to people with known infection. Sexual activity should be avoided until the lesions have healed.

Cytomegalovirus Mononucleosis

A syndrome virtually identical to that produced by Epstein-Barr virus (EBV) can be caused by the related virus cytomegalovirus (CMV). This virus is ubiquitous; more than 90 percent of homosexually active men attending STD clinics have evidence of previous infection with this virus, as do approximately 65 percent of heterosexual adults attending these clinics. Most of the time no symptoms are present, but patients may develop any of the symptoms of infectious mononucleosis (see below).

After infection, this virus may persist in saliva, semen, cervical secretions, urine, and blood. Thus, CMV mononucleosis is transmitted by sexual activity including vaginal intercourse or oral–genital sex (especially if semen is swallowed) and also by blood transfusions.

CMV has been linked epidemiologically to Kaposi's sarcoma and was initially discussed as one of the candidate viruses involved in the epidemic of AIDS. Following CMV mononucleosis there may be an alteration in the ratio of T-helper to T-suppressor cells, but this usually returns to normal in six to twelve months (see Chapter 9).

Pregnant women may carry CMV in the genital tract and it may spread to the infant during pregnancy or birth. Congenital CMV infections occur in about 1 percent of births in the United States, and this infection may produce nervous-system damage (including retinal damage) and developmental retardation. It may be carried in breast milk as well as the blood serum and saliva.

CMV mononucleosis is diagnosed by the typical findings of mononucleosis in the absence of a positive blood test for EBV antibody, as well as a rise in antibodies to CMV in the blood serum. There is no universally applicable treatment for cytomegalovirus infections. Prevention is achieved by judicious limitation of sexual partners. A vaccine, however, is under development.

Donovanosis

Donovanosis, another ulcerating condition of the genitalia, previously known as granuloma inguinale, is relatively rare. In the past several years only about seventy cases have been reported in the United States. The pathogen, *Calymmatobacterium granulomatis*, or *Donovania granulomatis*, is somewhat difficult to culture, but the organism can be seen under microscopic examination of stained pus or tissue taken from a lesion. The disease has a relatively long incubation period, which may last up to several months following contact. Small pimples, or nodules, on the penis, the vulva, the mouth, or the tongue ulcerate. Some of these ulcers may be fleshy and covered with an unpleasant-smelling exudate. Ulcers are chronic and may also occur on the skin over the abomen or the pelvis or around the anus. Rarely lesions may spread to the bones and other organs. Early lesions may mimic lymphogranuloma or chancroid.

Diagnosis is made by identification of the organism in a small tissue sample, and treatment is with antibiotics, including the tetracyclines, ampicillin, streptomycin, gentamicin, trimethoprim-sulfamethoxazole, and other agents. These drugs are generally prescribed for three weeks. Donovanosis is a reportable STD.

Donovanosis is not readily transmissible in that only a minority of contacts actually develop the disease. Very little is known about prevention of this disease, but sexual activity should be avoided in the presence of lesions. Condom use may reduce the risk of transmission.

Epididymitis and Prostatitis

Although epididymitis and prostatitis may occur in men at almost any age and may not be due directly to a sexually transmitted infection, they can result from a sexually transmitted organism. The epididymis is that portion of the seminal tube closest to the testicle, which may become infected with a variety of organisms. *Chlamydia tracho-matis* and the organism of gonorrhea are among the most frequent causes of infection of the epididymis, but recent studies suggest that other bacteria normally found in the feces (*E. coli*) may cause this infection in homosexual men who practice anal intercourse.

Diagnosis is made by inspection. A urine culture or direct aspiration of the epididymis may also be helpful. Treatment of this condition involves antibiotics appropriate for the particular infecting organism. Very little is known about the transmissibility and prevention of this infection.

Prostatitis is inflammation of the prostate gland, which sits at the base of the bladder in men. Many organisms, including *E. coli*, klebsiella, or streptococci, cause prostatitis. Diagnosis is made by physical examination by a physician as well as by examination of urine and any secretions that may result from massaging the prostate gland. A doctor can feel the prostate gland by digital examination of the rectum. When inflamed with acute prostatitis, the gland is tender to the touch. Treatment is based on the particular diagnosis and includes antibiotics. Chronic prostatitis may follow any episode of acute prostatitis, and the cause of this condition is usually difficult to identify.

It is not clear whether acute bacterial prostatitis is sexually transmitted. Nonbacterial prostatitis, however, has been associated with some sexually transmitted pathogens, including *Trichomonas vaginalis* (see Chapter 4), but the causal relation to prostatitis of this and other organisms, including *Chlamydia trachomatis* (see Chapter 3) and genital mycoplasmas, remains controversial. No known preventive measures exist.

Genital Warts

Genital warts are extremely common and account for 3 to 4 percent of the visits to STD clinics. Physicians are not required to report cases of genital warts to public-health authorities in the United States, but data from Great Britain, where reporting is required, indicate that this STD has increased dramatically during the past fifteen years.

Genital warts are caused by a virus, the human papilloma virus, which is related to the virus responsible for the common wart that affects other areas of the body. Up to twenty-five different types of human papilloma virus (HPV) have been recognized, and it is likely that more strains of this virus exist. It is unlikely for genital warts to be inoculated from those on the finger or the hand. Genital warts are believed to be sexually transmissible, but the very long incubation period (three months to one year) often makes the tracing of sexual partners difficult.

A curious phenomenon exists among homosexual men with anal warts in that the presence of anal warts is several times more common than penile warts. If genital warts were highly infectious sexually, one would expect penile warts to develop in partners of men with anal warts when anal intercourse is practiced. This does not appear to be the case, however. This phenomenon may be due to the long incubation period of this virus. It is possible that the virus responsible for anal and genital warts inhabits the anal area and is then activated or implanted during anal intercourse.

Genital and anal warts affect both men and women. The vulvar area, the clitoris, and the area around the urethra, as well as the lips of the vagina, are commonly infected in women who may also have anal warts, especially when anal intercourse is practiced. Men may have warts on the underside of the penis, around the head of the penis, and under the foreskin if uncircumcised. Some people develop warts inside the opening of the urethra, which can result in painful urination. Warts may develop on the tongue following oral sex, but this happens rarely.

Warts are usually soft and fleshy and may have a cauliflowerlike appearance. In some people the lesions become extensive and may coalesce and form large masses. In most cases these lesions are not painful, but they are relatively unsightly and may interfere with sexual activity. These lesions are known to increase in size in pregnant women and in people who develop immune-suppressing diseases.

Women with vulvar warts may also develop warts or wartlike lesions on the cervix. Symptoms are rarely caused by these lesions, which are usually detected on examination with an instrument known as a colposcope. The colposcope allows for direct visualization of the cervix by the doctor, who may note the presence of small, flat wartlike lesions. In some cases the vulvar or penile lesions may become quite enlarged and may look like symptoms of cancer.

A long history of genital warts may slightly increase the risk of uterine or genital cancer in women, but the precise relationship has not been defined. Two of the papilloma viruses that cause genital warts have recently been implicated as causes of cervical cancer.

People with genital warts often have other sexually transmitted diseases, including gonorrhea, urethritis, or syphilis. In most situations a physician will routinely screen for these other diseases even if warts are the only symptom.

Babies born to mothers with extensive vaginal or vulvar warts may develop small warts on the larynx, or vocal cords. Adequate treatment of the warts during pregnancy can help prevent this problem. Occasionally some women undergo cesarean section if warts are extensive.

Diagnosis of genital warts is usually made by the physician on the basis of a physical examination. There are no specific diagnostic tests. If anal warts are present, the doctor will probably perform an anoscopic, or proctoscopic, examination, which involves inserting a well-lubricated tube into the anus, allowing visualization of the mucous membrane of the rectum. This is necessary because in some situations there may be internal warts in the rectum that may "seed," or inoculate, external lesions. Rectal warts can be treated through a proctoscope. Pap smears are usually obtained in women to rule out the presence of an early cancer. Occasionally a biopsy of the wart itself is taken if other diseases such as tumors are suspected.

Treatment of genital and anal warts is difficult because of the tendency of these warts to recur even after apparently successful treatment. Many preparations, as well as several surgical approaches in severe cases, have been used to treat genital warts. Weekly topical applications of podophyllin are widely used and administered to destroy tissue infected with a wart virus slowly, but the tissue around the wart itself may become irritated. For this reason, podophyllin must be washed off after about four to six hours. This treatment is effective in about 60 or 70 percent of cases, but may not be effective in extensive lesions. If podophyllin is applied in large amounts to very extensive warts, it may be absorbed through the skin and cause nerve damage, depression of some blood elements, and liver damage. Podophyllin should not be used in pregnancy. Other topical applications may be used by your physician, including the drug 5-fluorouracil. Some warts do respond to vaccine treatment made from the patient's own wart, but this technique has not been universally accepted.

The three surgical techniques most frequently used to treat urogenital warts are electrocautery, cryosurgery (freezing), and surgical excision of the large lesions. Very recently, the use of laser surgery has been introduced. In this technique, a high-powered light source destroys the wart directly. In all of these treatments, recurrence may follow and there may be some discomfort in the post-surgical period. Treatment before the lesions become extensive is likely to be less painful and more effective.

Patients under treatment for anal or genital warts should refrain from sexual intercourse until the lesions have disappeared and should continue to use condoms to prevent subsequent transmission to sexual partners.

Infectious Mononucleosis

Infectious mononucleosis, or glandular fever, is caused by the Epstein-Barr virus (EBV), a virus that resembles the viruses of herpes and chicken pox. Infectious mononucleosis is extremely common, especially in adolescents and young adults, although it is sometimes diagnosed also in children. The Epstein-Barr virus usually is found in saliva and spread by intimate kissing. It can also be spread by way of shared drinking and eating utensils. Epstein-Barr virus is also known to cause Burkitt's lymphoma, a cancer of the lymph glands, as well as a nose and throat cancer.

These malignant complications are most common in Africa and China and are less common in America and Europe.

This illness has an incubation period of one to two months. Some patients are infected with EBV with few or no symptoms. Most people, however, develop a common symptom complex that includes fever, sore throat, and swollen glands, as well as enlargement of the spleen and the liver and swollen eyelids. Jaundice, rash, and anemia occur less frequently. Possible abnormalities in liver function may resemble those seen in hepatitis. Fatigue and an increased need for sleep are also characteristic of infectious mononucleosis.

Diagnosis of infectious mononucleosis is made by several different types of blood tests. Infected people have blood counts that are usually abnormal with an increased number of white blood cells and lymphocytes, some of which may appear atypical. The presence of a variety of specific and nonspecific antibodies is also considered in the diagnosis.

The most common blood test for infectious mononucleosis is the "monospot test." Positive results indicate the presence of nonspecific so-called heterophile antibodies typically found in this infection. It is important to note that monospot tests and other blood tests for mononucleosis are most accurate four to six weeks after the infection begins. Blood-test results may show up negative if performed too early. Tests for specific EBV antibodies performed early in the illness are usually accurate. Nonspecific and monospot tests remain positive for about a year after infection; EBV-antibody tests may remain positive forever.

There is no specific treatment for infectious mononucleosis. Some people will require bed rest due to severe fatigue, while others carry out their normal activities, provided they have several extra hours of sleep. Very rarely, patients with extremely swollen tonsils sometimes require a short course of steroids to reduce swelling. Patients whose spleen is enlarged should not participate in body-contact sports, to prevent or minimize the risk of rupturing the spleen. Over 99 percent of patients with infectious mononucleosis recover without complications, and splenic leaks or ruptures are rare.

It is quite common for people with mononucleosis to also become genuinely infected with "strep throat" due to the streptococcus. Penicillin or erythromycin is generally used to treat the streptococcal infection during mononucleosis, but these drugs have no activity against the EBV virus itself. Ampicillin or amoxicillin may also be used, but have been associated with a very high frequency of producing a rash.

Prevention of infectious mononucleosis is generally limited to avoiding intimate kissing with those who are known to have this disease or those who are recovering from it. Active secretion of the virus in the saliva may last for several months or longer after the onset of infection.

Lymphogranuloma Venereum

Lymphogranuloma venereum (LGV) is a relatively uncommon, reportable sexually transmitted disease in the United States. Between 125 and 250 cases are reported annually. Most of these cases have been reported from New York, Atlanta, and Washington, D.C.

LGV first manifests as a papule, or pimple, on the outside of the penis one to three weeks after contact with an infected person. The pimple gradually forms a shallow ulcer, but this ulcer or skin lesion is not usually noticed in the vagina or on the cervix by women. Several weeks later, large swelling develops in the lymph nodes on the affected side. This is the symptom that usually brings patients to seek medical advice. Sinuses may develop over the swollen glands and chronically drain. These swollen lymph glands, generally present in the groin, are tender. Symptoms of LGV may also include fever, chills, malaise, headaches, joint pains, and generalized lymph-node swelling. Lymph nodes in the neck of people who develop LGV as a result of oral–genital sexual contact may become extremely swollen and tender. Enlarged lymph nodes in the genital area may obstruct the normal drainage of lymph channels from the external genitals and cause the labia or the scrotal tissues to swell. LGV may also produce an inflammatory abscess in the rectum in men or women who practice anal intercourse, and proctitis may result in scarring and constriction of the rectum. LGV may also cause urethritis.

There may be an asymptomatic carrier state, but this is not well understood. Effects on the fetus or infant born to an infected mother are not well known.

Diagnosis of LGV is generally made if antibodies to the organism are found in the blood or with a special skin test. LGV is caused by specific strains of the organism *Chlamydia trachomatis* (discussed under Urethritis and elsewhere in this book). In specialized laboratories these organisms can be cultured from samples of fluid from the swollen lymph glands, but this test is not widely available. Aspiration of the swollen glands is usually performed to rule out the presence of other bacteria that may cause the swelling.

Treatment of lymphogranuloma venereum is usually with sulfa drugs or tetracyclines and is prescribed for at least three weeks. Methods of prevention are not well understood, but early diagnosis and treatment and limiting sexual activity until treatment is complete should help control the spread of this disease.

Molluscum Contagiosum

Molluscum contagiosum is an imposing name given to the pearly-white skin lesion caused by the molluscum contagiosum virus. These lesions may appear as single papules or as isolated papule clusters anywhere on the body in children, but usually on the genitals in adults. They vary in size from about two to three millimeters (requiring a hand lens to see them) to one centimeter. They tend to have pinpoint depressions in the center.

Molluscum contagiosum is thought to be transmitted by close contact in children and by sexual activity in adults. Adults with genital lesions of this disease often have other STDs as well.

Diagnosis is made by inspection of the typical lesion. A smear of the contents of a lesion may reveal intracellular inclusions. The lesion is then either mechanically removed, with a needle or a curette, or chemically treated with retinoic acid or liquid nitrogen. The emptying of the contents of the lesion tends to result in its ultimate cure. Occasionally, these sores heal by themselves. There is no specific medication for this infection. Prevention is limited to condom use and avoidance of sex with affected individuals.

Skin Infestations (Crab Lice and Scabies)

Infestation with crabs has become more frequent among sexually active people in the last ten years. (With parasites or insects we speak of *infestations,* rather than *infections* as with bacteria, viruses, or fungi.) Sexual intercourse, however, is not the only way in which crabs may be transmitted. All that is really needed is close physical contact. The crab louse is a tiny insect that measures about one-tenth of an inch. Its four legs resemble the pincers of a crab and allow the crab louse to adhere tightly to hair shafts, usually at their base.

Pediculosis, or infestation with lice, occurs at different body sites, depending on the species. The crab louse, *Phthirus pubis,* is best adapted for the hair in the pubic and perianal areas, the usual sites of infestation. However, these insects may occasionally be found under the arms, in the beard or the mustache, and rarely on eyebrows or eyelashes.

Crabs survive only on humans, and they generally die within one or two days away from their host. Thus, lice left on clothing or bed sheets cannot survive for more than one or two days. Crab lice are relatively slow-moving and tend to remain in the pubic area. Mating is frequent among adult insects. Adult females lay several eggs each day directly on the hairs. The little white egg cases, or nits, can be easily distinguished with a hand lens or a microscope, but when viewed directly they resemble pearly-white flakes (like dandruff) that cannot be removed easily. Adult insects live for about thirty days.

Symptoms begin roughly two to six weeks after contact with the adult crab louse. Some people develop no obvious symptoms. However, itching in the pubic area is usually the major symptom, caused by the injection of saliva when the louse bites the superficial layers of the skin to feed on blood from the capillaries. This itching may be due to direct irritation or to an immunologic response to the saliva. It usually results in rather profound scratching, which further increases the irritation and redness of the area. Occasionally, these insects spread to the thighs and produce similar symptoms there. They frequently produce small blue spots in the skin that may help confirm the diagnosis. These spots are due to the partial digestion of the red blood cells that remain deposited in the superficial layers of the skin.

Crab lice generally require intimate body contact for transmission. Occasionally, however, they do transmit by way of shared towels, bedding, or undergarments. This is one contagious disease that may potentially be spread by way of toilet seats and other inanimate objects. It should be remembered, however, that the insect dies within a day or two away from the human host. Head lice—commonly found in schoolchildren—generally do not infest the pubic area, and pubic lice rarely spread to the scalp area.

Treatment of crabs is simple and effective. A variety of pediculicides is available to eradicate the insect. The most commonly prescribed treatment is with lindane, also known as a gamma benzene hexachloride (Kwell and Scabene). Other preparations are available as over-the-counter medications, including A-200 Pyrinate, Cuprex, Li-Ban, R&C shampoo or spray, RID, Triple X, and Vleminckx. These medications should be applied to the affected area after a warm bath. Kwell lotion is left in place for twelve to twenty-four hours and then washed off. Some physicians recommend two applications at eight-hour intervals. The egg cases, which are generally emptied of their insect contents by the pediculicide, can be removed with a fine-toothed comb. One application is usually sufficient, but a second course of treatment one week later may be recommended by your physician.

Lindane-containing compounds (e.g., Kwell) should be used with caution during pregnancy, and none should be used in excess amounts. Side effects are usually limited to skin irritations, but irritation of the nervous system can occur in young children if too much medication is used. Consult your physician for persistent problems with lice. Occasionally, itching may persist for several days after treatment as a result of the pediculicide, but then disappear promptly. Recently worn clothing, sheets, pillowcases, towels, and other possibly infested items should be washed in hot water and dried at high-heat settings.

About 30 percent of crab-lice-infested patients attending STD clinics have other sexually transmitted diseases as well. Many physicians, therefore, perform routine screening tests for other STDs on their patients with crab lice.

Prevention of this infestation is limited to the joint treatment of sexual partners and avoidance of sexual contact with infested people.

Scabies is a disease of the skin caused by a microscopic mite that is similar to the one that causes mange in dogs. Scabies is not transmitted exclusively by sexual contact; it can be spread by any close contact with an infested individual. It can be found within families and frequently in children. The female mite typically burrows into the superficial layers of the skin, where she lays her eggs. These eggs hatch and both male and female immature insects develop within the skin. They may cause a tiny pimple.

Scabies may occur in any area of the body and characteristically produces itching that may be more severe at night. The skin of the pubic area, the penis, or the scrotum may be infested in men; however, the external female genitals are rarely infested with scabies.

Diagnosis is usually made by inspecting the lesions and by finding a burrow of an adult female. The burrow or adjacent irritated lesions are scraped off and then examined in a drop of mineral oil under a microscope. The presence of adult mites, eggs, or insect droppings confirms the diagnosis.

Treatment of scabies is with topical scabicides including lindane (Kwell), sulfur compounds, or crotamiton. These preparations should be applied as directed; excessive use may cause skin irritation. Babies born to mothers who have used Kwell excessively during pregnancy may develop irritation of the nervous system (e.g., seizures). Recently worn clothing and used bedding should be washed in hot water or boiled.

Prevention of scabies is limited to avoidance of close contact with infested people.

Traumatic Lesions

Sores or irritations may occur on the penis or the vulva as a result of sexual activity. These conditions are not infections per se, but may contribute to infection. Heavy sexual intercourse, masturbation, mechanical injury from zippers or other objects, and the application of some substances to the genitals may also irritate the skin of the penis or the vulva. Those who develop sores, or abrasions, as a result of trauma should give a detailed account of the likely reason for injury so that the physician is not misled by a lesion that may mimic other diseases that are sexually transmitted. Usually the shape of traumatic ulcers, or lesions, is less distinct than those caused by sexually transmitted infections.

Traumatic sores or wounds can become secondarily infected with bacteria that are normally present in the genital area. The lymph glands that drain the area may become swollen and make diagnosis difficult; the complex of genital sores plus swollen lymph glands may suggest several infectious diseases. In these cases your physician will attempt to rule out the more common STDs such as syphilis and herpes.

Treatment of traumatic genital lesions depends on the nature of the condition and the type of infecting organisms, if any. In general, these lesions heal by themselves unless seriously infected. Some physicians apply an antibiotic-steroid ointment, which may allow for more rapid healing of certain lesions. The use of steroids or cortisone creams or ointments in the presence of infected lesions without the simultaneous use of antibacterial medication may only worsen the condition.

Prevention of traumatic lesions is limited to adequate lubrication during sexual activity and care to avoid irritation to the genitals.

Other skin diseases may also produce lesions on the genitalia and need not imply the presence of any sexually transmitted disease. For example, psoriasis, eczema, sebaceous cysts, and other types of dermatitis may occur in the genital area.

11 / Preventing STDs

In the past, physicians and health authorities invested a great deal of energy in the prevention of sexually transmitted diseases. In the first half of this century most cases of venereal disease were syphilis or gonorrhea, and most prophylactic or preventive approaches were directed against these infections. Much of the impetus for prevention came from the military, where STDs were frequent causes of lost productivity.

During World War I, the military established many "VD stations" in cities where large numbers of servicemen were billeted. These stations were charged with the responsibility of providing postexposure prophylaxis to soldiers, who were required to report for treatment after each episode of sexual intercourse. These stations provided a routine that was effective (albeit a bit unpleasant) against infections due to gonorrhea and syphilis.

This procedure involved urinating, then washing the genitals in warm water and liquid soap poured on by an attendant. The genitals were examined for discharge or sores. In addition, a silver solution was instilled into the urethra, which was then held closed for five minutes by the soldier. After this solution was released, the penis was then rubbed with a calomel (mercury-containing) ointment and wrapped in gauze. The soldier was instructed not to urinate for four to five hours. Severe penalties for failing to report sexual activity included docking of pay, relief of duty, and, in some cases, court-martial.

During World War I, having a venereal disease was a military offense, and soldiers with syphilis and gonorrhea were termed "sexual offenders." The military exacted considerable punishment for soldiers caught, and the virtues of chastity were preached as a part of basic training. At one point, venereal camps were proposed for sexual offenders. Despite, or perhaps because of, these severe measures, only about 20 percent of those who had sexual contact actually reported for treatment. In a sense, the fear of discovery was worse than the fear of developing the disease itself.

Fear of venereal diseases has rarely been an effective means of prevention. Sexual activity is a basic aspect of life, and sexual expression is a major human need.

During World War II, the Pro-Kit was introduced, and it was also used by civilians during and after the war. The Pro-Kit contained a sulfa drug, calomel, and a supply of condoms.

Other chemicals, including mercury bichloride, silver solutions, and soap and water, have been used as post-exposure prophylaxes for decades. A preparation of orthoi-odobenzoic acid called Progonansyl has been useful in the prevention of gonorrhea and syphilis. This compound has been used by prostitutes, among others, and when applied frequently to the vagina it dramatically reduces the risk of transmitting gonorrhea to sexual contacts. Many women, however, develop vaginal irritations and have found it too troublesome to use routinely.

With the introduction of effective antibiotics against gonorrhea and syphilis, it became easier, in many cases, to treat a widely established infection than to prevent one. Today, with the multiplicity of STDs, the increasing resistance of gonococci to penicillin and similar antibiotics, the epidemic proportion of such STDs as herpes, and the appearance of an apparently lethal sexually transmitted disease in the form of AIDS, renewed efforts toward prevention must be made.

METHODS OF PREVENTION

LIMITING SEXUAL PARTNERS

There are no specific sexual practices that are responsible for transmission of STDs in the absence of the causative organism. However, the risk of contracting an STD associated with any particular sexual practice increases with the number of different sexual partners. When two partners are involved in an exclusively monogamous sexual relationship and both are free of any sexually transmissible infectious agent, there is no risk of STDs developing in either partner. The couple need not limit the frequency of sex nor refrain from specific sexual practices under these obviously safe circumstances.

The concept of "safe" sex implies limiting the number of one's sexual partners. Each time the number of sexual contacts increases, one significantly increases the risk for acquiring an STD. If one member of a couple has outside sexual relations, then both partners are at an increased risk of acquiring an STD. Obviously, sex with professional prostitutes, male or female, is likely to be associated with a greater risk of acquiring STDs.

A recent *New York Times* article has reported the possible end of the sexual revolution. It appears that having multiple sexual partners is going out of style among homosexuals as well as heterosexuals. Fear of herpes and AIDS most likely has contributed to this decline, but other social factors are probably also involved.

Public awareness of genital-herpes infections, fanned a great deal by press reports, is on the minds of many young sexually active people. It is very difficult, if not impossible, to select partners who have never been infected with herpes simplex virus. A recent report suggests that uninfected partners of those with known genital herpes are at very low risk of acquiring this infection if the couple refrains from sexual activity during the presence of any active lesions. Having a frank discussion of STDs and the history thereof between sexual partners is thus very important. An open and supportive attitude will help reduce fear, embarrassment, and guilt, as well as the diseases themselves.

Sexually active gay men are at particular risk of acquiring sexually transmitted diseases. The risk dramatically increases with an increase in the number of sexual partners. Gay men with four or more different sexual contacts per month are considered at high risk of contracting STDs, while those with one or fewer sexual partners per month are considered at low risk. Since frequent and anonymous sexual contact is common and accepted in the gay community, and since many of the organisms responsible for STDs may be present at various sexual sites without producing any symptoms, it is easy to understand how, once introduced, any sexually transmissible agent can disseminate rapidly through the gay community. Given the frequency of asymptomatic carriers of many infecting organisms, some specific sexual practices have been associated with a significant risk of STD. Anal intercourse (active or passive), oral–anal sex, and fist fornication are activities associated with high risk. These activities have been associated with an increased risk of hepatitis B, hepatitis A, enteric infestations and infections, and AIDS. Oral–genital sex is associated with an intermediate risk; kissing, mutual masturbation, and other body contact are associated with a lower risk of contracting an STD.

For gay men, safe sex involves knowing one's partner and his sexual history and limiting one's contact with new or multiple partners to those activities associated with low risk—for example, mutual masturbation. Even high-risk activities (with the exception of fist fornication) can be safe when practiced with a single longtime partner.

Gay men are also advised to wash the genital area before and after sex to reduce the risk of contracting syphilis, gonorrhea, and possibly urethritis. Washing alone, however, is not an effective preventive. Rectal douching, or using enemas, prior to sex or after, may, in fact, increase slight trauma and bleeding of the rectal surface and thereby increase the transmissibility of such diseases as hepatitis B.

In addition, if amoebas are present, they also may be washed into the rectal area during an enema and may actually increase the risk of transmitting amebiasis. There is no way of making oral–anal sex safe except by limiting one's activity to a single partner in a monogamous relationship in which both partners are known to be free of STDs.

The National Coalition of Gay Sexually Transmitted Diseases Services (NCGSTDS) has a detailed pamphlet entitled "Guidelines and Recommendations for Healthful Gay Sexual Activity," which is available from P.O. Box 239, Milwaukee, WI 53201-0239. Additional information about AIDS is available from the National Gay Task Force's AIDS Crisis Line at 1-800-221-7044. Most cities have gay health referral services or clinics with personnel trained to provide information and care to gay men.

HYGIENE

Soap is an effective inhibitor of the spirochete that causes syphilis. In general, washing of the male and female genitalia before and after sexual activity is a reasonable means by which to maintain general cleanliness and lower the number of sexually transmissible organisms present externally. General washing, however, does not affect organisms located inside the vagina or on the cervix and does not reach any urethral surfaces. Although recommended, soap and water do not completely eliminate the risk of contracting an STD.

Vaginal douching may reduce the number of trichomonad organisms and yeastlike fungi present, but frequent douching may result in irritation and drying of the vaginal mucous membranes, which may, in turn, result in irritation during intercourse.

BARRIER METHODS

The condom has been in existence for more than four hundred years. Originally made of animal skins or intestines, today these prophylactics are made of latex rubber. Condoms are regulated and tested by the Food and Drug Administration and are reliable, safe, and effective in the prevention of STDs. ("Lambskin" condoms are made from the large intestine of lambs and are not tested in the same manner and, therefore, are not necessarily proven reliable in preventing STDs.) The condom is also an effective contraceptive.

It is very difficult to prove in large-scale studies the effectiveness of condoms in preventing specific sexually transmitted diseases. Obviously it is difficult to determine uniform compliance with condom usage during any study. Nonetheless, there is a great deal of evidence suggesting that this choice will prevent or reduce the spread of gonorrhea, syphilis, and the agents of nonspecific urethritis. Herpes simplex virus infections and genital warts may also be preventable with a well-fitted condom but only at those sites that are in fact covered by the condom sheath. A recent in-vitro study suggests that the condom can prevent transmission of herpes simplex virus and *Chlamydia trachomatis* from one partner to another.

The effectiveness of the condom in reducing sexually transmitted diseases depends upon its uniform use. It must be used for each and every sexual contact and it must be properly placed and properly removed. There can be no unprotected genital contact during foreplay. All of these restrictions may seem to inhibit the spontaneous act of lovemaking and diminish the moment of passion. However, those who routinely use the condom during lovemaking will dramatically reduce the risk of developing an STD.

Homosexually active men who practice rectal intercourse with multiple partners are urged to use this prophylactic device. It is highly likely that most of the anally transmitted infections can be completely prevented with the use of condoms.

The diaphragm has been used primarily as a contraceptive, but many of the foams, jellies, and creams that are used with the diaphragm or alone may have some protective activity against STDs. Many of these products have some inhibitory activity against many sexually transmitted organisms. Some of these include Conceptrol, Delfen, Gynol II, Ortho-Creme, Ortho-Gynol, Emko Because, Emko foam, Koromex vaginal jelly, Ramses contraceptive vaginal jelly, Encare, and Semicid. These agents are marketed as contraceptives, and most of them contain the spermicide nonoxynol-9 in varying concentrations. This agent in high concentrations will inhibit the growth of the gonococcus within one minute after exposure.

These contraceptive products are not sold for the express purpose of preventing STDs, but with regular use they have some prophylactic effect, especially with a diaphragm. The use of these products cannot replace any of the methods mentioned above and are in no way guaranteed to prevent all STDs. They have no proven activity against herpes simplex infections, although laboratory tests suggest that they may have some activity against yeastlike fungi and the trichomonad organism.

ANTIBIOTICS

Antibiotics are extremely effective in the treatment of many venereal diseases, especially gonorrhea, syphilis, and chlamydial urethritis. It seems logical that these drugs would also be effective as prophylactic measures in the prevention of STDs. In fact, for an individual who infrequently engages in sexual activities that are high risks for transmitting STDs (for example, sex with prostitutes or occasional homosexual contacts), some studies suggest that prophylactic treatment with tetracycline or a related drug may be effective.

However, when sexual contacts and potential exposures to STDs are many, frequent use of antibiotics for prevention will inevitably increase the resistance of the microorganisms to the antibiotics. This has the net effect of reducing the effectiveness of antibiotics in treating sexually transmitted diseases, as well as many other types of infection. In addition, frequent use of antibiotics increases the likelihood of the user experiencing sensitization reactions to the drugs. And finally, since more than one STD may be present following any given contact, the use of one prophylactic antimicrobial agent might not eradicate all of the infections.

Self-treatment with leftover antibiotics may mask symptoms that might otherwise be easily identified and treated properly by your physician. An insufficient dose of antibiotics may only increase the microorganisms' resistance to the drug without actually killing them, thus making a final cure more difficult to achieve.

CONTACT TRACING

Contact tracing has been the mainstay of venereal-disease control efforts on the part of public-health departments. This process involves a frank, confidential discussion and disclosure of one's recent sexual contacts. For the most part this type of tracing has involved syphilis and gonorrhea. Named sexual partners are contacted confidentially by nonjudgmental public-health workers and are then urged to seek treatment, even if there are no symptoms present. Although this approach may result in treating some people who have been exposed but not infected, most, but not all, STD experts attest to the success of this treatment in reducing the spread of STDs.

SELF-EXAMINATION

People engaging in sexual activity with new or multiple partners should become comfortable with self-examination. The genitals should be examined frequently for the presence of unusual sores or lesions, which should be seen promptly by a physician. Waiting for lesions to go away only delays prompt therapy and heightens anxiety. As with lesions of genital-herpes infections, for example, the maximum benefit from the new antiviral ointment occurs when the drug is used within the first few days of infection. Waiting for several days or weeks will limit the effectiveness of any antiviral drug for this disease.

Gay men should examine their anus with a finger in the shower to be aware of any changes in this area. Some men periodically examine their anal area with a mirror. This may allow for early detection of anal warts, fissures, or other lesions.

CHECKUPS

Frequent checkups by your private physician or health clinic are strongly encouraged. Many STDs exist for a long time without producing symptoms and can be detected only by special cultures and examinations. The frequency of these examinations depends upon the number of different sexual partners. Highly sexually active people with multiple partners should be checked monthly for the presence of nonsymptomatic sexually transmitted diseases. Individuals who have less frequent activity or fewer partners should be checked perhaps every three or six months.

In general these screening tests involve blood tests for syphilis and cultures for gonorrhea from the sites of sexual exposure. In men a thin swab is inserted in the tip of the penis; the sample is then cultured on appropriate media. It generally takes three days to obtain the results of this test. Similar swab samples can be taken from the cervix, the rectum, and the throat.

Gay men should receive cultures of the pharynx, the urethra, and the rectum for detecting gonorrhea and blood tests for detecting syphilis. It is not always feasible for STD clinics to actively search for the presence of gastrointestinal parasites in a routine fashion. These tests are time-consuming, expensive, and often negative. However, those who believe they have been exposed or who are at high risk of developing enteric infection should request a detailed parasitic examination and culture.

You should certainly report to your doctor the presence of any symptoms in the genital or rectal area that might be associated with any STD. Until your examination, you should avoid sexual activity, in order not to spread a possible STD. You should become familiar with the signs and symptoms of STDs, and you should feel comfortable talking to new partners about your sexual history. Encourage them to communicate their sexual history to you.

When an STD is diagnosed and treatment is prescribed, it is very important to take the medication as directed. The symptoms that brought you to the doctor in the first place disappear very quickly, but the organism may persist for much longer. Its eradication and cure may require the full course of treatment. Medications should not be saved for administration at a later time; many become ineffective or may even become harmful after long periods of storage.

VACCINES

The future holds much potential for the development of safe and effective vaccines against STDs. A highly effective vaccine against hepatitis B is available. All high-risk people, especially gay men, should be screened for the presence of antibodies to hepatitis B (and hepatitis A). Susceptibility to these infections may be determined by the lack of antibodies in the serum to these organisms. If antibodies to hepatitis B are lacking, gay men and others at high risk should receive the hepatitis-B vaccine. This vaccine is administered in three doses, the first two at a monthly interval, the third six months after the first injection. This vaccine is safe and has been associated with only a few side effects, including mild fever and local tenderness at the injection site. There has been no evidence that the hepatitis-B vaccine is associated with the transmission of AIDS. The AIDS-associated virus is inactivated by the process used to produce hepatitis-B vaccine. A new vaccine made as a result of genetic engineering is currently under study.

In addition, vaccines against gonorrhea, genital herpes, and syphilis may be available within the next few years.

STD HOTLINE

The STD Hotline is a telephone service (maintained by the American Social Health Association) that provides toll-free information for anyone concerned about STDs. This hotline will also make referrals to physicians or health-care providers in your area who are trained and interested in the diagnosis and treatment of STDs. The hotline telephone number is 1-800-227-8922; in California 1-800-982-5883.